Ophthalmic Plastic Surgery

SMITH'S PRACTICAL TECHNIQUES IN

Ophthalmic Plastic Surgery

Frank A. Nesi, M.D., F.A.C.S.
Associate Clinical Professor of Ophthalmology and Otolaryngology,
Co-Director, Oculoplastic Service,
Kresge Eye Institute,
Wayne State University School of Medicine, Detroit, Michigan;
Chief, Oculoplastic Surgery,
Department of Ophthalmology,
William Beaumont Hospital, Royal Oak, Michigan

Kevin L. Waltz, M.D., O.D.
Eye Surgeons of Indiana,
Indianapolis, Indiana;
formerly Assistant Professor of Surgery,
Southern Illinois University,
Springfield, Illinois

with 281 illustrations in 72 plates by
Virginia Hoyt Cantarella, A.M.I.

with the collaboration of
John Siddens, M.D.

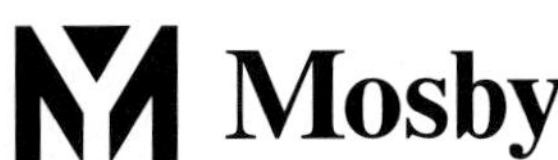

St. Louis Baltimore Boston Chicago London Madrid Philadelphia Sydney Toronto

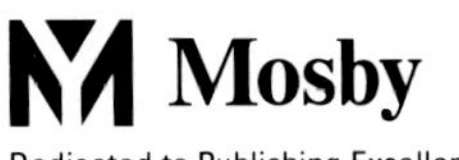 **Mosby**

Dedicated to Publishing Excellence

Publisher: George Stamathis
Editor: Laurel Craven
Assistant editor: Lauranne Billus
Project manager: Mark Spann
Production editor: Stephen C. Hetager
Manufacturing supervisor: Betty Richmond
Designer: David Zielinski

Second Edition

Printed in the United States of America

Mosby-Year Book, Inc.
11830 Westline Industrial Drive
St. Louis, Missouri 63146

ISBN 0-8016-6355-5

94 95 96 97 98 UG/MV 9 8 7 6 5 4 3 2 1

Dedicated to the memory of our mentor and friend, Byron C. Smith, who laid the foundation upon which we carve our initials; and to our wives Karen and Rhonda, without whose unselfish support and encouragement we would not have finished this task

PREFACE TO THE SECOND EDITION

During the preparation of this book my friend and mentor, Byron C. Smith, tragically died. For many months I was unable to confront the completion of this our last project together. Finally, with the encouragement of my wife Karen, my friend Virginia Cantarella, and many other friends and colleagues, we completed our task. I would also like to thank Dr. John Siddens, who helped to write, edit, and complete this task.

Once again we have attempted to update the techniques and details of a small number of procedures that we found useful in our practices. For those seeking more in-depth knowledge of a subject or a procedure not included in this book, we suggest our two-volume text, *Ophthalmic Plastic and Reconstructive Surgery,* also published by Mosby.

The explosion of knowledge in the past decade in the field of ophthalmic plastic surgery, the novel procedures and technique modifications currently being used, and the interest in the regional anatomy of the eye have made the task exciting.

A bibliography has been added. We have attempted to update those procedures that we still use and add newer ones. Once again we thank innovative surgeons for their ideas.

In spite of the recent proliferation of similar books, requests for our original text are constant and numerous. We hope that this book will help those with an interest in ophthalmic plastic and reconstructive surgery.

Frank A. Nesi

PREFACE TO THE FIRST EDITION

The preparation of this book was stimulated by our desire to update the technical details of a limited number of surgical procedures that we use frequently. Most of the operative methods were originated by others. The simple drawings and descriptive, concise text provide the details of the surgical approach to a number of frequently encountered abnormalities. The details and modifications are depicted and described in accordance with the methods we currently use.

We admit that it is much easier to draw diagrams of our operations than it is to perform the same procedure on living tissue. As in any other artistic endeavor, the results are dependent on the skill and artistic ability of the surgeon. It is beyond the scope of this book to alter these attributes in any individual surgeon. The suggestions contained in this publication are meant to crystallize the technical details and minimize the possibilities of complication and failure.

We are grateful to all those responsible for the original contributions to the field of ophthalmic plastic surgery. Had it not been for their originality and generosity, it would have been impossible to compile the contents of this book. In addition, we are grateful to all those responsible for our training and to those responsible for stimulating us to contribute additional knowledge to the field. Daisy Stilwell shall always be remembered for her many fine drawings that have proven helpful to Virginia Cantarella in the finalization of her artistic accomplishments in this book. We wish to thank Virginia Cantarella for her artistic ability and her many helpful suggestions. Finally, we appreciate the efforts of those hospitals, clinics, referring physicians, nurses, technicians, and all others responsible for our accomplishments.

Byron C. Smith
Frank A. Nesi

CONTENTS

Ophthalmic Plastic Surgery

CHAPTER 1

EVALUATION OF THE PATIENT

The preoperative evaluation of the patient about to undergo ophthalmic plastic or reconstructive surgery should begin with a consideration of the patient's attitude toward and expectations about surgery. The surgeon should give a candid appraisal of the anticipated results of surgery and should speak with sensitivity about that which is certainly an important matter for the patient—his personal appearance. This is of primary importance in establishing a good relationship with the patient and avoiding future difficulties. It is essential that the patient's expectations of the surgical results approximate reasonably achievable goals for the surgeon.

Preoperative photographic documentation of the patient is an integral part of the initial examination. We use a Polaroid camera in the office and routinely order 35-mm color slides and 5 × 7 black and white photographs to be taken prior to surgery.

A complete ophthalmic examination should be performed on every patient, regardless of the type of case. A corrected visual acuity is obtained. If indicated, visual field testing is performed by tangent screen or Goldman-type perimetry. In an unresponsive patient, examination of the pupils may indicate an afferent pupillary defect and therefore a monocular optic nerve lesion. (In a traumatic case, a paralysis of the iris or iris sphincter may result from a traumatic rupture.) An efferent pupillary defect is signified by a poor response to light directly or consensually and may indicate a compressive or traumatic lesion of the third nerve.

An external examination will reveal asymmetries of contour that may be within normal limits, as well as eyelid malpositions, lack of lid tonicity, cutaneous defects (scarring), or globe malposition (enophthalmus or exophthalmus). These abnormalities should be pointed out to the patient preoperatively. Baseline exophthalmometry measurements should be performed when indicated.

Slit-lamp examination of the conjunctiva can reveal cicatricial inflammation and injury from chemical or thermal burns, Stevens-Johnson syndome, pemphigoid, or an infectious process. As sequelae of these, scarring and deformity of the lids with entropion and trichiasis may result. The lacrimal ducts may be ablated, producing a dry eye. Small tumors of the lids and periorbita should be noted and suspicious lesions excised with clean surgical margins. The medial canthi should be carefully examined because of the dire consequences of late excision in this area.

A motility examination done at near and far in the cardinal fields of gaze is useful, because extraocular muscle imbalance is often associated with congenital defects, traumatic injury, or orbital tumors. Quantification done preoperatively not only may reveal the extent of ocular involvement but also may provide a baseline for postoperative evaluation.

Direct and indirect ophthalmoscopy following dilatation is also useful in revealing congenital defects and traumatic injury. Fundus abnormalities must be noted and documented preoperatively, because they may have a bearing on postoperative results.

The lacrimal system should be evaluated by the performance of secretory and excretory tests. A Schirmer No. 1 test to measure reflex and basic secretion should be performed first. Following the instillation of anesthetic solution, the basic secretors should be tested alone. Primary and secondary dye tests should then be performed to test the excretory mechanism. This testing is essential not only in cases of epiphora but also as a baseline in ptosis and blepharoplasty surgery, in which a slight overcorrection may cause a dry eye syndrome.

The ophthalmologist performing plastic or reconstructive surgery should use the expertise of related specialists. For example, personally reviewing the radiographs with the radiologist enhances the clinical information gained from the variety of radiographic techniques available. While plain films of the facial bones and skull may reveal the obvious fracture or foreign body, polytomography in coronal, submental vertex, or sagittal planes can document what are otherwise merely clinical suspicions. High-resolution computed tomography (CT scan) in axial, coronal, and third-dimensional projections are evaluated. Density measurement techniques of the CT scan, particularly when combined with orbital A-scan ultrasound, provide considerable information on the nature and pathology of a lesion. Magnetic resonance imaging (MRI) studies have become an excellent technique for detecting orbital diseases; they provide soft-tissue studies superior to CT imaging. Vascular and hemorrhagic lesions, as well as the extent of demyelinization, can be better studied because of MRI. The apex is no longer the safe harbor of orbital pathology. Tumors and vascular abnormalities of the orbit or cranium presenting with orbital signs may also require cerebral angiography of the external and internal circulation to document full anatomic features of the feeding and draining blood supply. The proper course of therapy may include the assistance of the neurologist, neurosurgeon, otolaryngologist, or maxillofacial surgeon in a cooperative surgical effort.

CHAPTER 2

ANATOMIC CORRELATION

To successfully perform plastic or reconstructive surgery of the eye or the ocular adnexa, one needs a thorough knowledge of orbital and eyelid anatomy. The success of split-thickness skin or composite dermis-fat grafting techniques depends on a knowledge of the microscopic anatomy of the integument. Performing ptosis surgery without having a thorough and precise knowledge of upper lid structures would be difficult if not impossible. The evaluation of orbital tumors or orbital trauma requires an understanding of the bony structures of the orbit with its inherent weaknesses and strengths. The complex structure of the medial canthal area with its enclosed lacrimal system must be understood for one to successfully perform surgery in this area.

The skin is composed of the epidermal layer, the dermal layer, and the subdermal fat (Plate 2-1). The hair follicles and sebaceous glands are contained within the deeper layers of the skin. To avoid inclusion of these follicles in a skin graft, one must make the graft sufficiently thin. Or, as in cilia grafting, the graft must be deep enough to include these elements, when this is the desired effect.

The full thickness of the skin refers to all of these layers, while split thickness refers to anything less than the full thickness.

Deepithelialization provides access to the dermis and fat layers of the skin, which can be used in dermis, fat, or composite dermis-fat grafts.

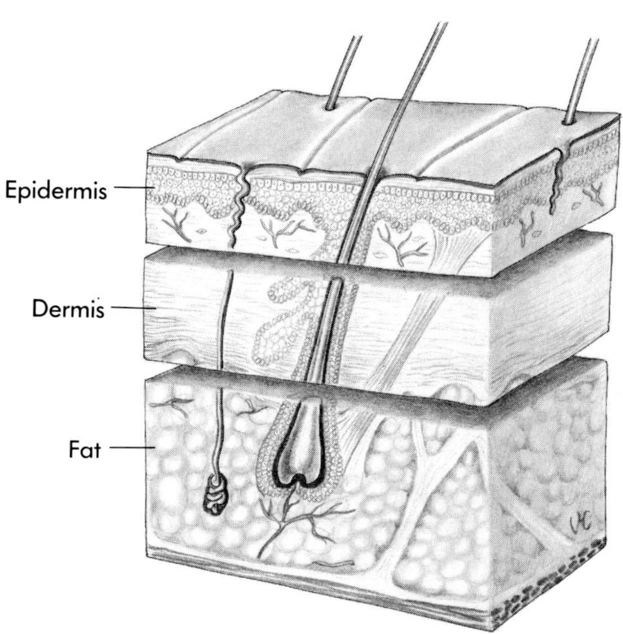

Layers of skin: epidermis, dermis, fat.

Superficially the lids are composed of a layer of thin, loose skin with little subcutaneous fat. In both the upper and lower lids are transverse folds (supratarsal creases), which in the upper lid correspond approximately to the top of the tarsus.

For surgical purposes the upper lid can be divided into five layers: (1) skin, (2) orbicularis muscle, (3) orbital septum, (4) levator aponeurosis and Müller's fibers, and (5) tarsoconjunctival layer (Plate 2-2). Underlying the skin is the orbicularis oculi, a continuous circular muscle that can be divided into orbital and palpebral parts, the latter of which is subdivided into preseptal (overlying the septum) and pretarsal (overlying the tarsus and more adherent) sections. At the lateral canthus, the pretarsal section from the upper lid joins that from the lower lid and forms the 7-mm lateral canthal tendon, which inserts on the lateral orbital tubercle. At the medial canthus, the pretarsal muscle divides into superficial and deep heads. The superficial heads unite to form the medial canthal tendon, which inserts at and nasal to the anterior lacrimal crest. The deep heads insert on the posterior lacrimal crest. Likewise, the preseptal muscle divides into superficial and deep heads, with the former inserting on the medial canthal tendon and passing to the posterior lacrimal crest, while the deep head inserts on the lacrimal diaphragm and aids in the functioning of the lacrimal pump.

The lacrimal excretory system is composed of the upper and lower puncti, with their corresponding canaliculi that descend vertically from the puncti for about 2 mm, and then course medially for 8 mm, uniting to form the common canaliculus. This empties into the lacrimal tear sac, which in turn communicates with the nose by means of the nasolacrimal duct (Plate 2-3).

The orbital septum originates from the superior orbital rim, to which it is strongly adherent. When the mesodermally derived levator muscle advances forward in its evolution, it pushes the orbital septum in front of it and then goes on to mesh with the pretarsal orbicularis fibers and insert in the lower tarsus. The space between the septum, which finally inserts on the levator aponeurosis, and the levator itself is called the preaponeurotic space and is generally filled with fat. This is an excellent landmark during external ptosis surgery. Posterior to the levator aponeurosis is the postaponeurotic space. This space separates the aponeurosis from the smooth muscle fibers of Müller's muscle, which inserts on the tarsus.

Finally, there is the tarsal layer, about 10 mm wide in the upper lid as opposed to 4 mm wide in the lower lid. Closely adherent to the tarsus is the conjunctiva. It is this close adherence, combined with the juxtaposition of the postaponeurotic space, that makes dissection of a tarsoconjunctival flap feasible.

The lower lid is analogous to the upper lid, but its structures are less well defined (see Plate 2-2). The principal difference is the retractor system. The retractor of the lower lid, in contradistinction to the well-defined levator muscle, is a fibrous extension of the inferior rectus muscle, the movement of which gives the lower lid its motility.

The retractor, originating from the inferior rectus muscle as the capsulopalpebral head, encapsulates the inferior oblique muscle. Anterior to it, the fibers unite as the capsulopalpebral fascia to insert on the inferior tarsal border but not into the orbicularis, and therefore the lower lid crease is poorly defined.

The septum fuses with the capsulopalpebral fascia below the tarsus. Therefore note that this plane is reached from the conjunctival side before the orbicularis septal plane is reached.

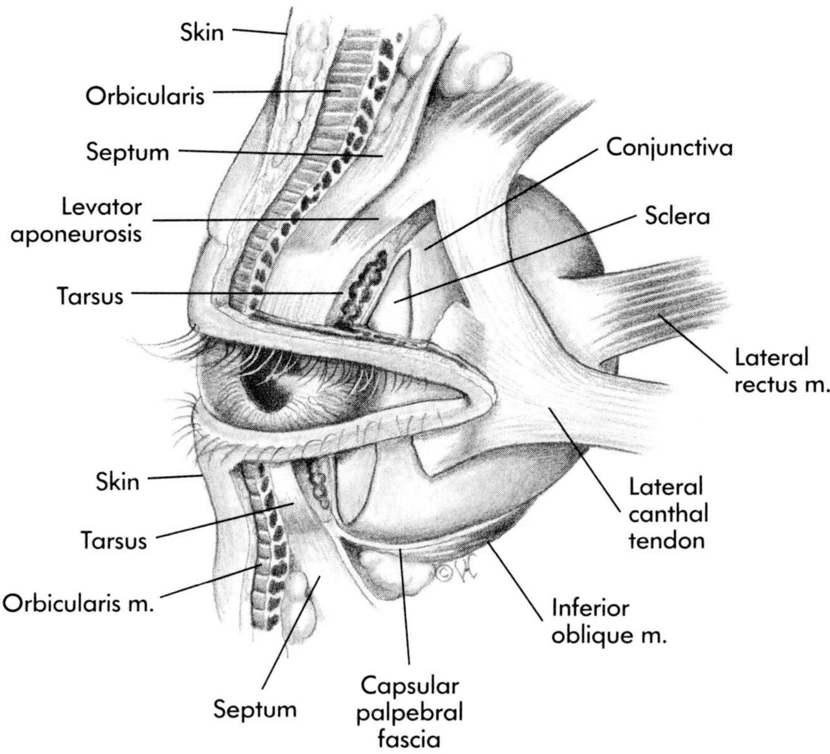

Anatomic layers of the upper and lower eyelids.

Anatomy of medial canthal area to show relationship between lacrimal excretory system and medial canthal tendon. Inset demonstrates canalicular system.

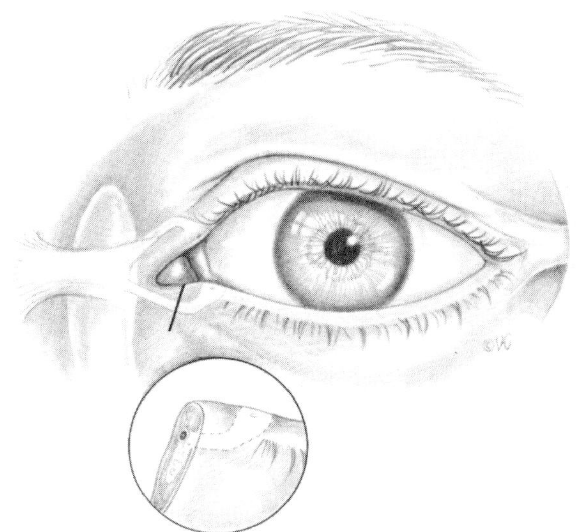

The orbits are generally described as four-sided conical structures, with the base forward and projecting medially toward the optic foramen. The base, or orbital rim, is outlined by strong bony abutments: the supraorbital arch of the frontal bone above, the zygoma and maxilla below, the zygoma laterally, and the frontal process of the maxilla medially. The walls of the orbit consist of relatively thin bone.

The orbit is further divided into four parts: the roof, the medial wall, the floor, and the lateral wall. The roof of the orbit is, for the most part, composed of the orbital plate of the frontal bone and posteriorly the lesser wing of the sphenoid (Plate 2-4, *A*). The pulley for the superior oblique muscle is lodged 4 mm behind the rim.

The medial wall, the thinnest of the orbital walls, is formed by the frontal process of the maxilla and the lacrimal bone, which together form the lacrimal groove (Plate 2-4, *B*). Just behind the posterior lacrimal crest is the extremely thin lamina papyracea of the ethmoids and finally the lesser wing of the sphenoid and the optic foramen.

The triangular orbital floor is formed by the zygomatic bone, the orbital process of the palatine bones, and, for the most part, the orbital plate of the maxilla, which is anterior to the infraorbital fissure. This is the area most frequently involved in blowout fractures of the orbital floor (Plate 2-4, *C*).

The lateral wall of the orbit is composed of the frontal process of the zygoma and the frontal bone anteriorly and the greater wing of the sphenoid posteriorly (Plate 2-4, *D*).

Plate 2-4

A, Roof of orbit.

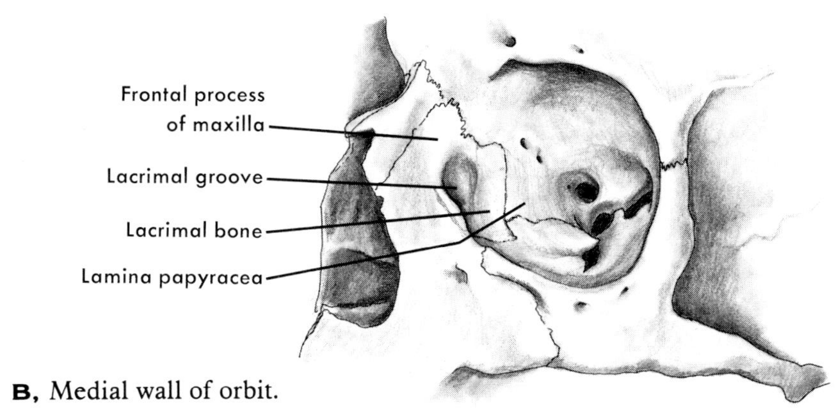

B, Medial wall of orbit.

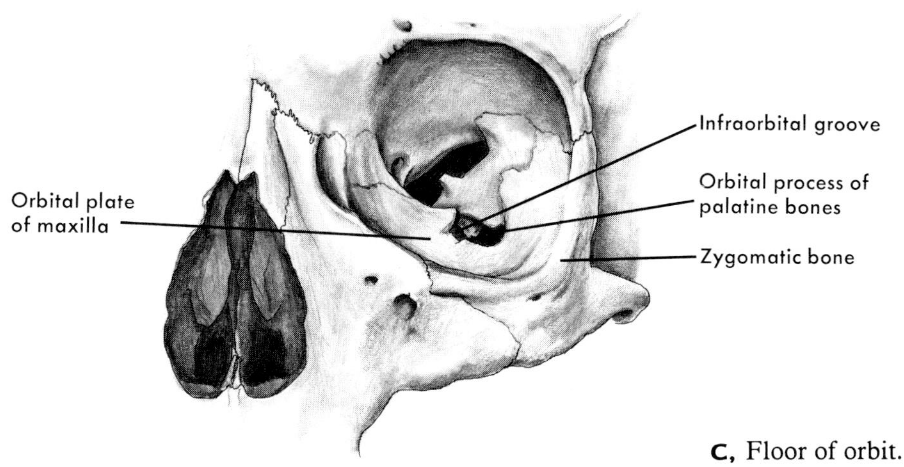

C, Floor of orbit.

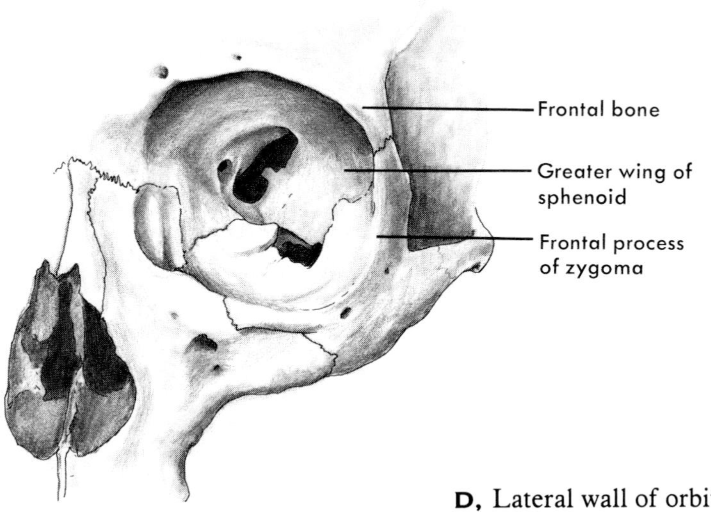

D, Lateral wall of orbit.

CHAPTER 3

SURGICAL PRINCIPLES

Although advances in the manufacture of surgical suture material, needle design and fabrication, and exquisite instrumentation have certainly increased the possibility of achieving acceptable results in all areas of surgery, including ophthalmic plastic surgery, there is no substitute for the skillful application of sound surgical principles and the sensible use of well-conceived surgical techniques in achieving successful surgical results. A precise knowledge of the regional anatomy, used to interrelate the various components of the ophthalmic complex, and judicious and gentle handling of tissue components are necessary to achieve successful reconstruction.

To achieve accurate apposition of adjacent tissue layers, the correct placement and tying of sutures are essential. An inaccurately placed or inaccurately tied suture can distort the tissue margins and result in a deepened or depressed scar.

To correctly place an appositional superficial suture, the wound edges should be everted. The suture should be inserted close to the wound margin and moved subcutaneously away from the margin edge. At the base of the wound, the suture should be turned and withdrawn in a similar fashion, to be inserted once again very near the edge of the opposite wound margin. The depths to which the suture is inserted on each side of the wound should be as equal as possible to prevent the formation of a depressed scar. The suture is then tied with multiple square knots and with sufficient tension to cause a slight upward puckering of the wound edges (Plate 3-1, *A*).

Placement of the suture too far from the wound edge will cause inversion of the skin margin and resultant increased cicatrization. If this suture is tied too tightly, the circulation will be compromised and a delay in the healing process will result (Plate 3-1, *B*).

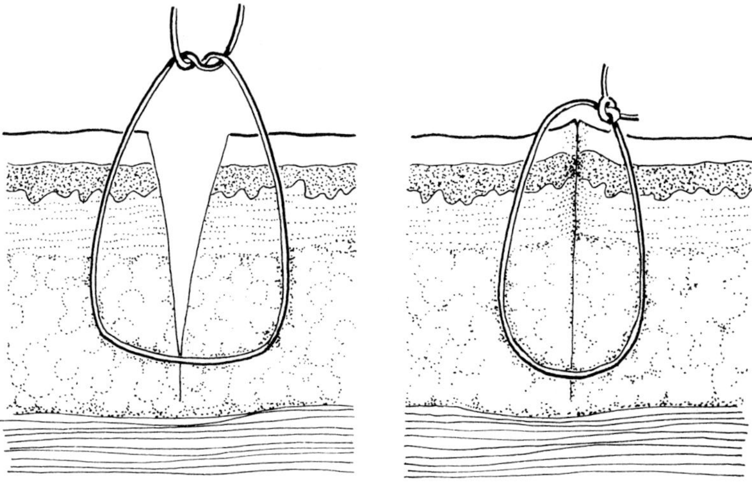

A, Correctly placed interrupted superficial closure: skin edges slightly puckered after tying.

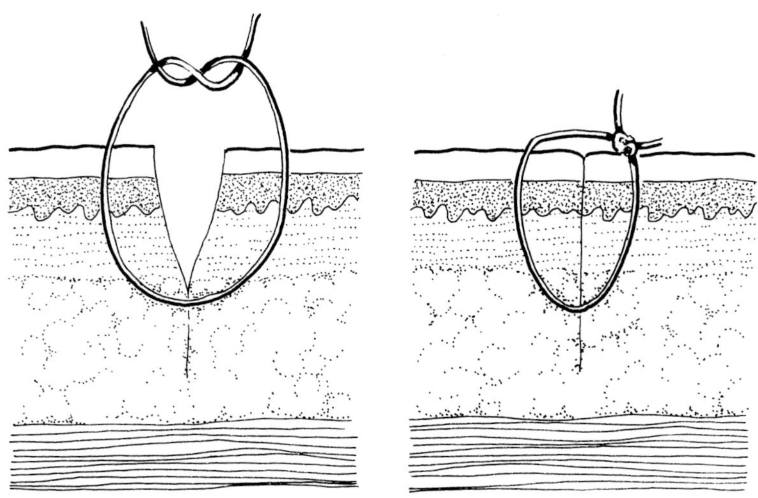

B, Incorrectly placed suture: suture too far from skin edges: inversion of margins when suture is tied.

An attempt should be made to close a deep wound by the placement of a suture as near as possible to the base of the wound. If the wound is too deep for the proper placement of a single superficial suture, the deeper layers should be closed by alternate methods, with the intent of eliminating surgical dead space and the possible contracture this may cause, as well as relieving the superficial sutures of undue tension.

By simply inserting a suture in the deep layers, drawing the needle toward the surface, and reinserting the needle downward in the opposite side of the wound, the surgeon may place a buried suture with its knot turned downward (Plate 3-2, *A*). As many as necessary of these buried sutures are placed to relieve the tension in the skin surface. Conventional sutures are then placed on the surface.

The same goal can be achieved with a figure-of-eight suture, although the effectiveness of this suture is limited by the difficulty of its proper placement. The advantage of a properly placed figure-of-eight suture is the lack of tissue reaction to the buried component, which is removed when the superficial portion is removed (Plate 3-2, *B*).

The end-on vertical mattress suture is also useful in eliminating dead space by closure of deep tissue. The peripheral support provided by the placement of this suture also produces a good apposition of superficial wound edges. When these sutures are used, they should be alternated with simple interrupted sutures, because they tend to suppress circulation. When this suture is inserted into the underlying fascia, good apposition can also be achieved with separated underlying tissue (Plate 3-3).

Plate 3-2

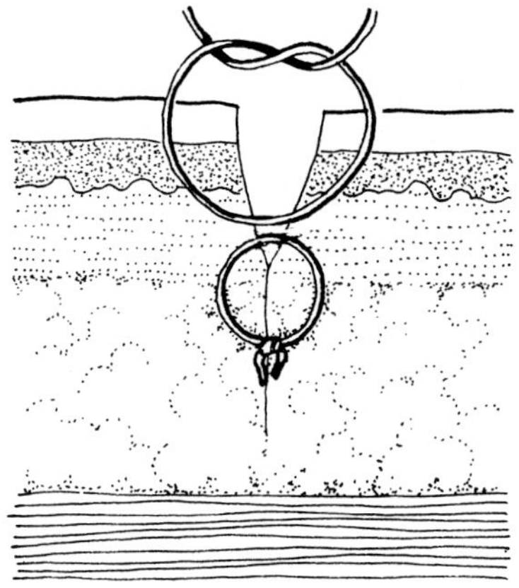 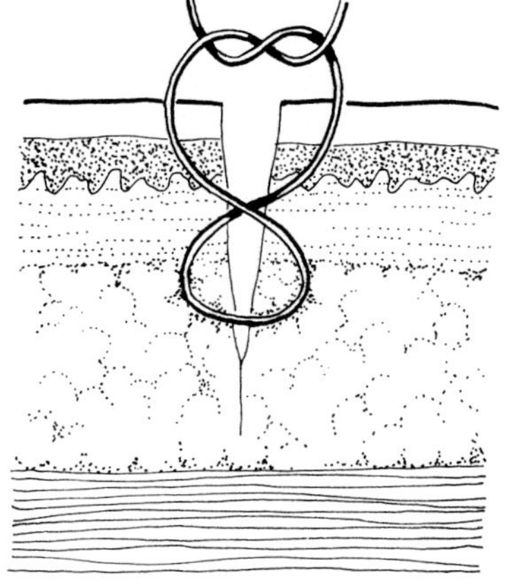

A, Buried suture used to close deeper layers. Syperficial layer closed with interrupted suture.

B, Figure-of-eight suture used to achieve same closure.

Plate 3-3

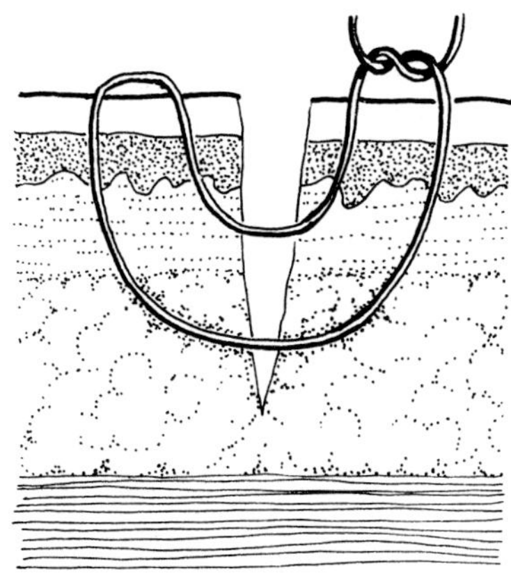 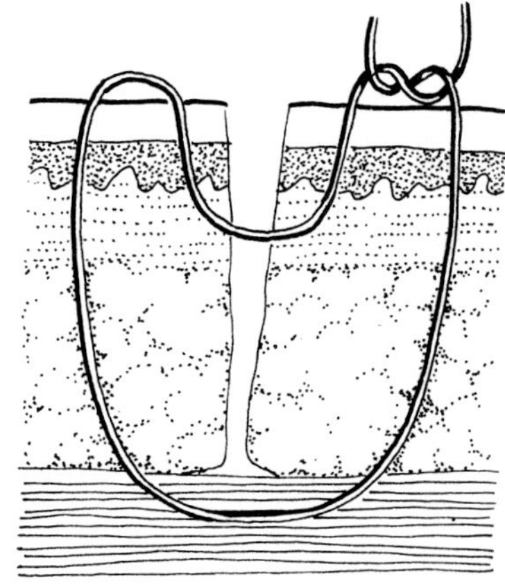

A, End-on vertical mattress suture used to eliminate dead space.

B, End-on suture used to bind superficial layer to underlying tissue.

For the closure of noncomplex lacerations a time-saving and effective technique is the use of continuous locking or nonlocking sutures. If care is taken to equalize the tension along the length of suture placement, this method can produce a satisfactory wound closure. One method of placement of a continuous locking suture is demonstrated in Plate 3-4. The surgeon must decide on the appropriate technique at the time of surgery.

An alternative method of wound closure is the use of permanently buried interrupted subcutaneous sutures. Absorbable suture material is used for this horizontally placed appositional stitch. Often the wound apposition obtained makes the placement of superficial sutures unnecessary and eliminates the possiblity of epithelialization of superficial suture tracts. This suture may be placed as a continuous subcuticular stitch (Plate 3-5).

An ingenious technique of suture placement, the near-far, far-near suture is inserted into the wound superficially, near its margin, drawn across the hiatus, penetrated deeply, and withdrawn some distance (5 to 10 mm) from the skin edge (Plate 3-6, *A*). The suture is then reinserted on the opposite wound margin at an equidistant point, placed into the deep tissue, from which it is withdrawn, and again drawn across the wound, to be withdrawn at a superficial point near the margin of the wound. The two-layered closure requires suture of sufficient strength to relieve the tension of the wound and facilitate its superficial closure (Plate 3-6, *B*). Interrupted sutures are then interspaced at 1-cm intervals (Plate 3-6, *C*). The interrupted sutures can be removed before the near-far, far-near sutures, which are generally left in place for 1 week. The wound is generally adhesively bound for several days to ensure continued wound apposition.

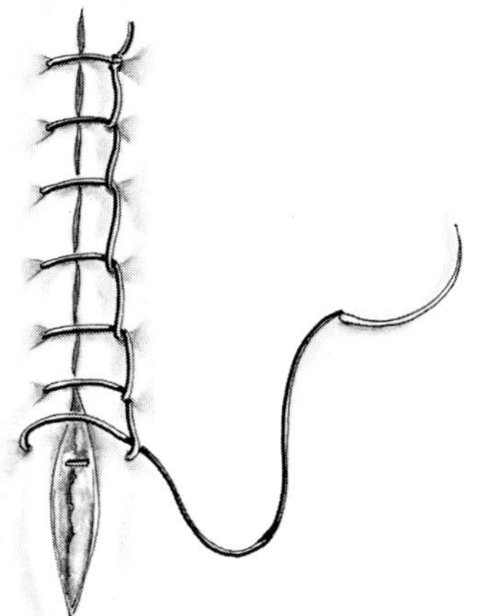

Continuous locking suture.

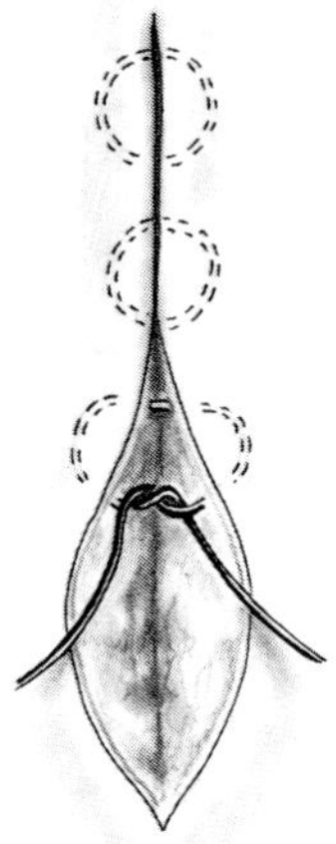

Interrupted subcutaneous sutures.

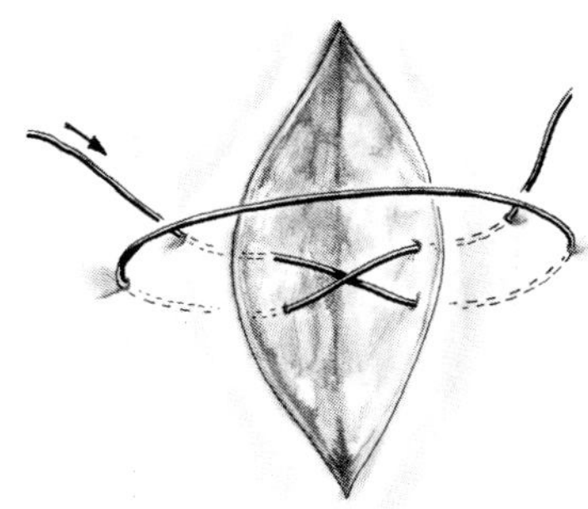

A, Near-far, far-near suture used to relieve tension.

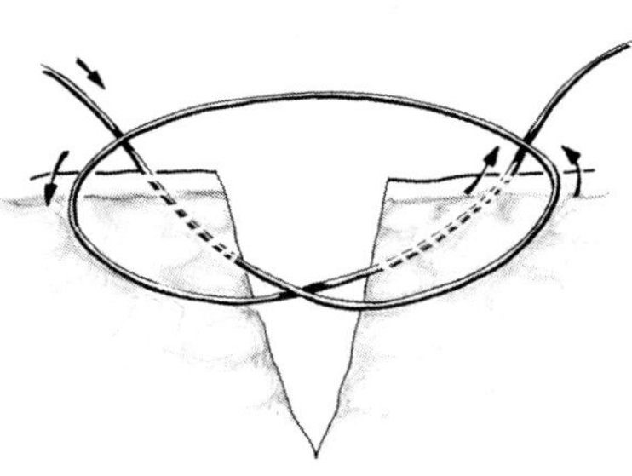

B, Directional course of near-far, far-near suture.

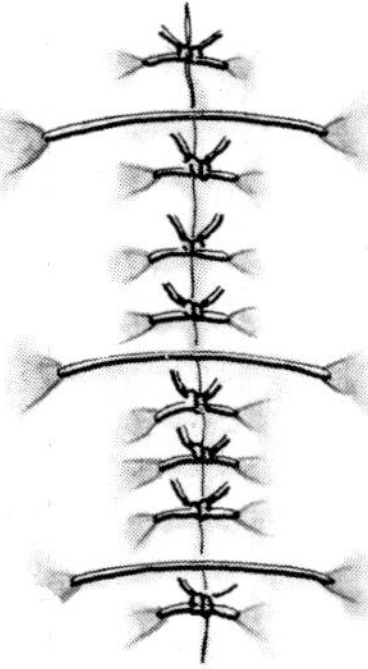

C, Placement of near-far, far-near suture interspaced with interrupted horizontal sutures.

USE OF FLAPS

Defects caused by traumatic injury or tumor excision that cannot be closed by direct apposition of severed tissue can be filled by various skin flaps. Skin flap design is based on the extent, type, and location of the area to be filled.

Sliding flap
(Plate 3-7)

In some instances it is possible to undermine the tissue in a subcutaneous plane adjacent to the wound margins for a sufficient distance from the wound edge to allow tension-free closure of the defect. By repeatedly drawing together the wound edges as the dissection proceeds, one can determine when the wound will close in a tension-free fashion (Plate 3-7).

Linear advancement flap
(Plate 3-8)

A simple linear advancement flap can be used to close a rectangular defect. Parallel incisions are made from the edge of the defect, sufficiently deep to include the vascular bed and up to 2½ times the width of the area to be filled. Care is taken not to compromise the circulation. The flap is gently dissected until it can be slid into the defect with minimal tension. Interrupted 6-0 silk sutures are used to close the wound.

If the length of the defect is greater than 2½ times its width, the advancement or transposition of the flap is delayed; that is, it is dissected and replaced into the donor bed for a period of 2 to 3 weeks to allow for longitudinal vascularization of the flap. At the end of this time, it is again dissected free and advanced into the recipient site (Plate 3-8).

Rotation flap
(Plate 3-9)

A rotation flap is created by incising a semicircular (curvilinear) pathway from the edge of the defect and carving a pedicle flap, again dissecting gently to include the vascular bed (Plate 3-9). The pedicle is then rotated to fill the defect. Suturing is simultaneously begun from both ends of the defect until a puckering of the curved aspect of the flap donor site is apparent. This area is then excised in a triangular fashion, and the triangle is closed with interrupted sutures.

Plate 3-7

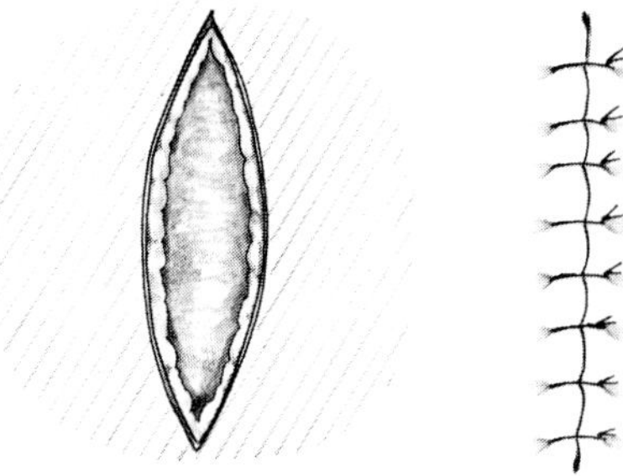

Wound margin undermined to
achieve sliding flap closure.

Plate 3-8

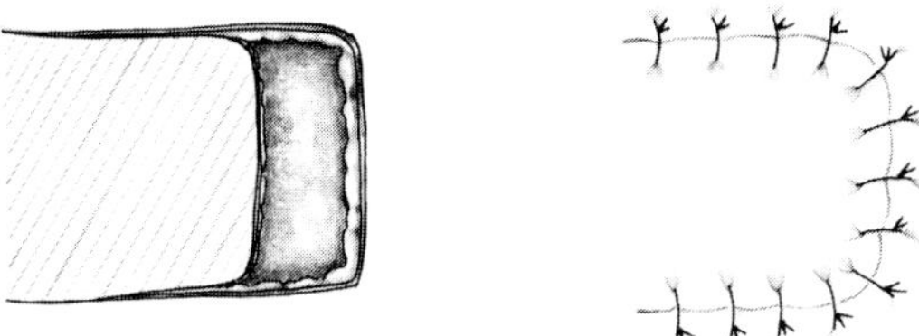

Simple linear advancement flap.

Plate 3-9

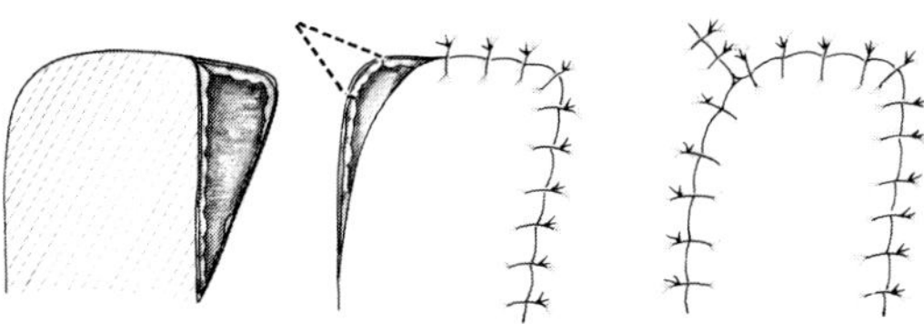

Rotation flap with triangle removed
to facilitate closure.

Combined sliding flap and advancement flap (Plate 3-10)

The techniques of using sliding and advancement flaps can be combined to fill a defect in which both sides of the wound need to be utilized for closure. With the previously described methods, the flaps are created, advanced, and sutured closed (Plate 3-10).

Transposition flap (Plate 3-11)

A transposition flap is used to close a defect in a nonadjacent area (Plate 3-11). Similar to the advancement flap, in that the flap must be delicately dissected and sufficiently thick to allow for an adequate vascular bed, this type of flap must also be gently transposed with delicate ophthalmic plastic instruments to ensure its viability. The donor site, if unable to be closed with simple undermining of adjacent tissues, may have to be filled with an advancement flap or possibly a free skin graft, to be modified at a later date.

Plate 3-10

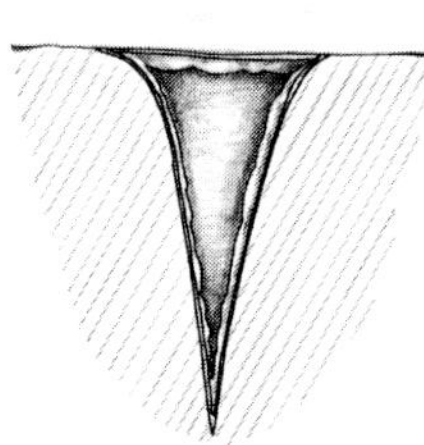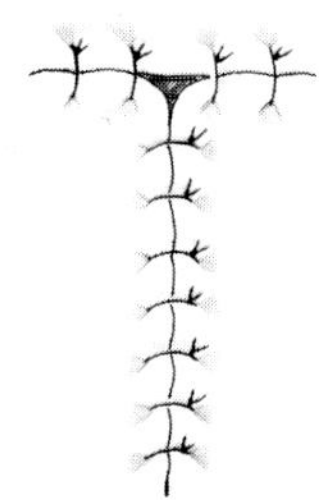

Combined sliding flap and advancement flap.

Plate 3-11

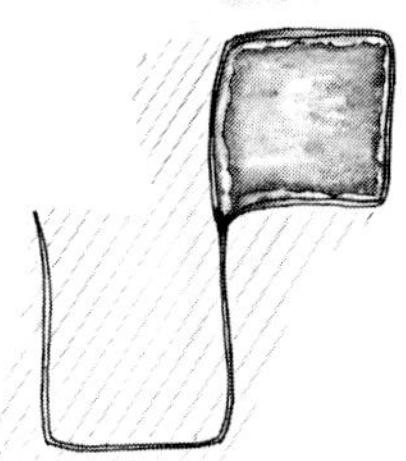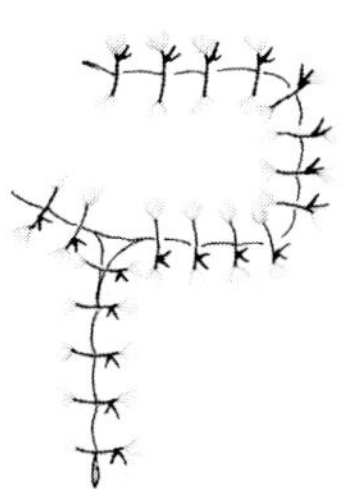

Transposition flap used to close nonadjacent defect.

Technique

(Plate 3-12)

Z-plasty is a procedure essential to any reconstructive surgeon. It is used to relieve lines of tension caused by a contracted scar. The retraction is released by transposition of skin flaps and excision of the underlying cicatricial tissue. The rotation of the skin flaps can lengthen the contracted area by up to one third of its present length.

The Z-plasty is begun by making a central incision through the scar. Two incisions are then offset 60 degrees from the ends of the central incision (Plate 3-12, *A*). While the assistant handles the skin flaps very gently to avoid necrosis, the surgeon gently dissects them free of underlying scar tissue, but deep enough to include a vascular supply (Plate 3-12, *B*). The resulting skin flaps are equal-sided triangles. Any remaining subcutaneous scar tissue must be completely excised. Failure to release all of the cicatricial bands will cause the scar to re-form and to recontract.

After meticulous dissection, the skin flaps are ready to be transposed (Plate 3-12, *C*). The flaps are transposed from the original Z configuration to something resembling a lightning bolt, thus lengthening the original scar (Plate 3-12, *A* and *D*). The incision is now closed with interrupted 6-0 mild chromic sutures (Plate 3-12, *E*). It is usually easier to close the incision at the base of the triangles first, progressing toward the apex.

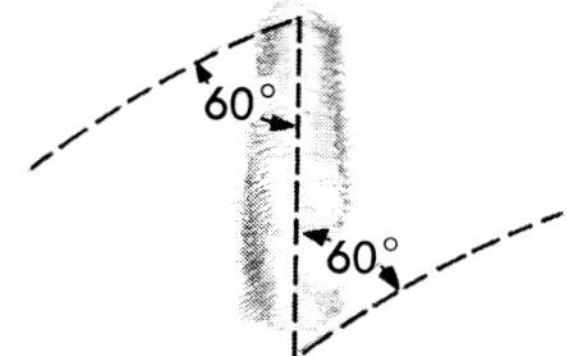

A, Central incision through line of traction, with arm lines offset at 60-degree angles.

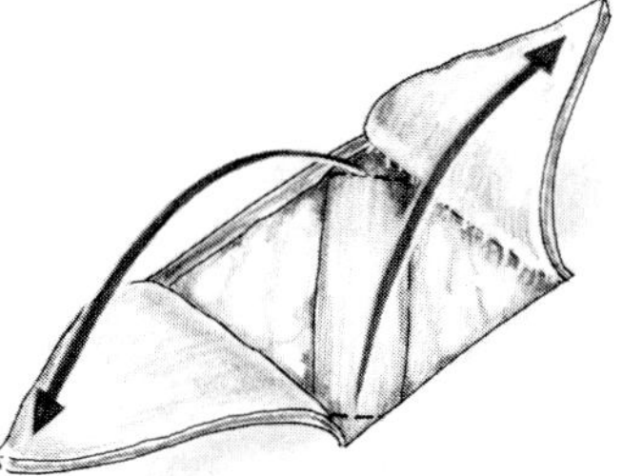

B, Flaps dissected free and elevated.

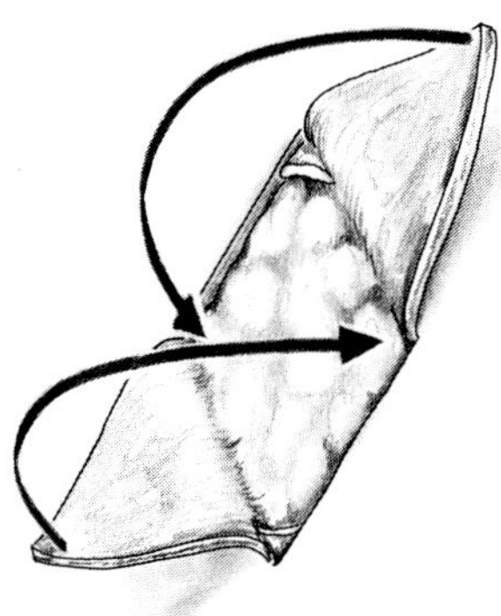

C, Fibrotic band excised and flaps ready for transposition.

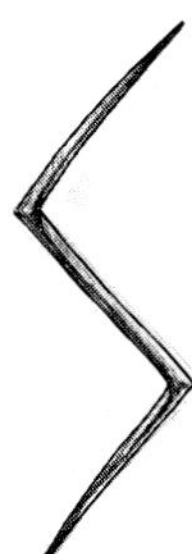

D, Flaps have been transposed.

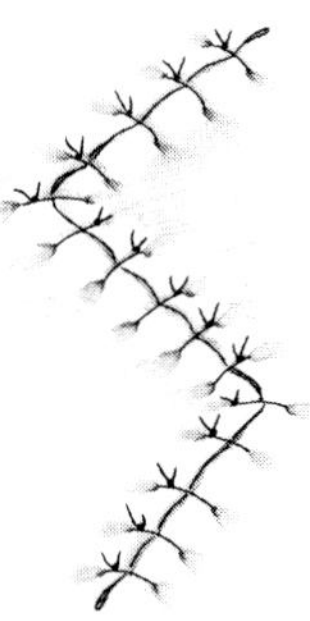

E, Flaps sutured into position.

Cicatricial band (Plate 3-13)

A cicatricial band causing vertical shortening of the upper lid (Plate 3-13, *A*) and resulting lid retraction and lagophthalmos can be corrected with a Z-plasty. The central scar is incised, and a tension-relieving incision is made on either end of the central incision (Plate 3-13, *B*). The flaps are dissected free, and underlying scar tissue is completely excised (Plate 3-13, *C*). Failure to completely excise the cicatricial tissue will produce a suboptimal result. The flaps are handled very gently to avoid any compromise of their blood supply. Cautery is kept to a minimum to avoid thermal contraction of collagen in the base of the incision.

The flaps are gently transposed from the original Z pattern into the lightning bolt configuration to vertically lengthen the lid. The incision is closed with interrupted 6-0 mild chromic sutures. A double-armed 4-0 or 6-0 silk suture is placed through the upper lid, including some tarsus, and a small cotton bolster is placed under the suture to prevent skin necrosis. The upper lid is placed on stretch with the silk suture by taping it to the cheek or suturing it through the skin and tying it over a cotton bolster (Plate 3-13, *D*).

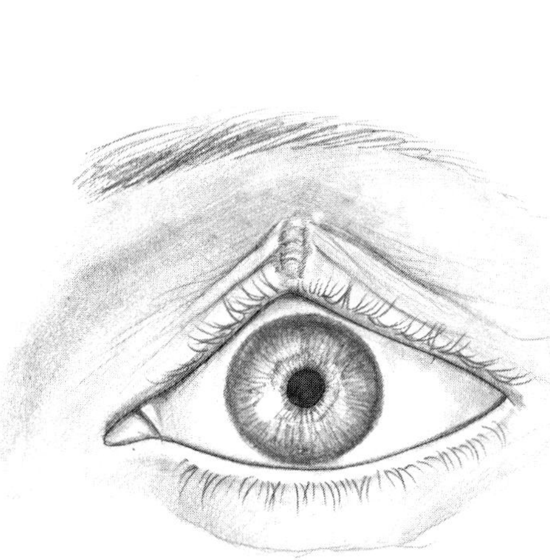
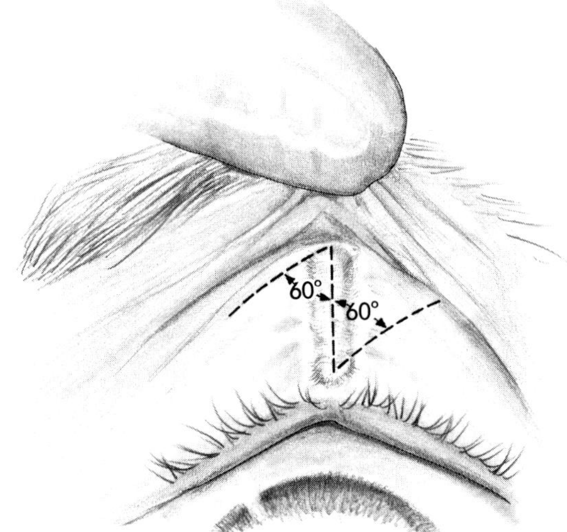

A, Cicatricial band causing vertical shortening of the upper lid.

B, Central line through scar, with arms offset at 60-degree angles.

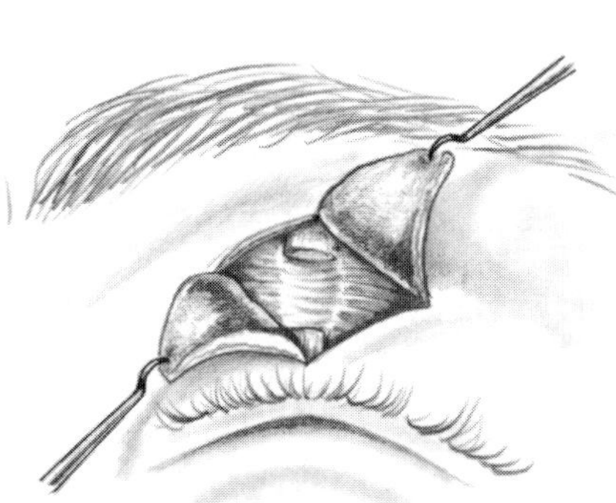
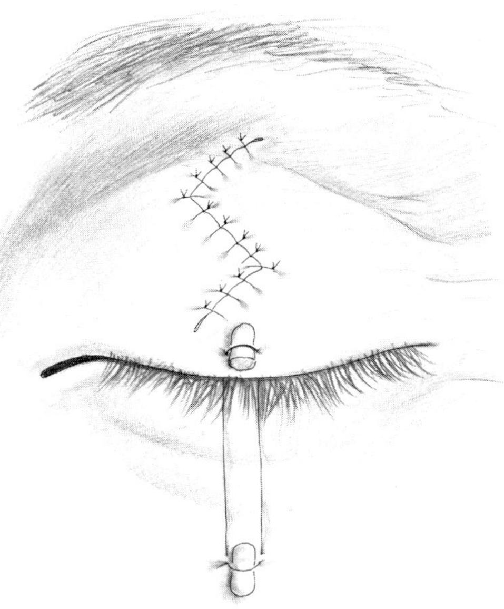

C, Fibrotic band excised and flap ready for transposition.

D, Flaps transposed and sutured into position with upper lid placed on stretch.

Multiple Z-plasties may be helpful for facial or brow scarring that is too pronounced for dermabrasion to be used alone. The technique follows the guidelines just described. The initial incision is made along the length of the scar, and multiple offset incisions are made on each side of the scar at 60-degree angles to the initial incision (Plate 3-14, *A*). The offset incisions are placed evenly. Their length is equal to the distance between the offset incisions.

The flaps are dissected, and underlying fibrotic tissue is completely excised. The triangular flaps are then transposed. They will virtually fall into place, if the underlying scar tissue has been adequately excised. Interrupted 6-0 mild chromic sutures are used to secure the flaps into position (Plate 3-14, *B*).

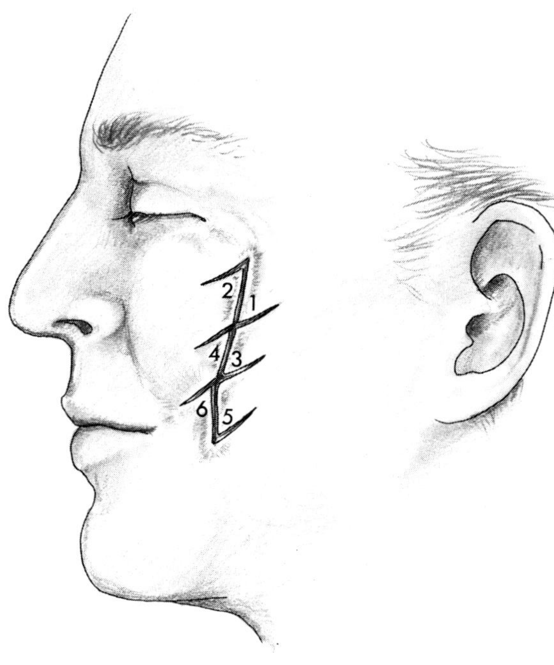

A, Multiple Z-plasty prepared.

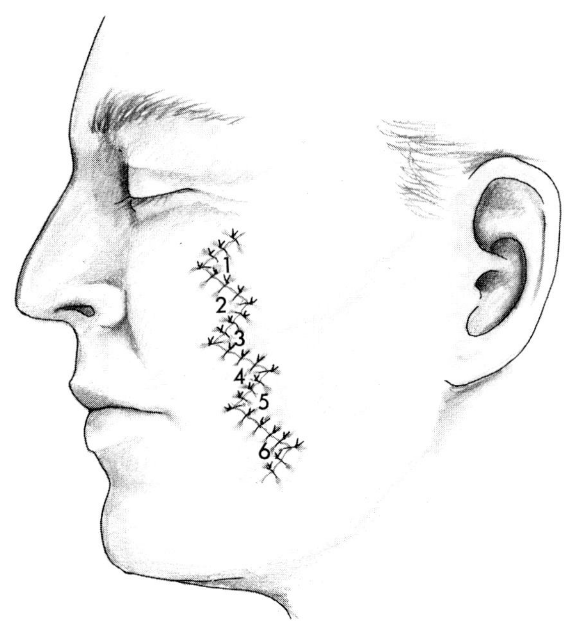

B, Flaps transposed and sutured into position.

A modified Z-plasty may be used to create a rotational skin flap at the lateral canthus to elevate or lower the lateral canthus and lateral lids. A 4-0 silk suture is placed through the lid margin of the contracted lid, and the lid is stretched. A subciliary incision through skin and fibrotic tissue is made 2 mm below the lash line and extended out to the lateral canthus. The incision is then turned medially, and the central portion of the Z is created, with the incision ending just before reaching the supratarsal crease. The Z is completed by incising laterally to outline a temporally based flap (Plate 3-15, *A*). After adequate dissection and excision of the underlying cicatricial bands, the upper triangular skin flap is transposed into the lower lid defect. The upper lid and the transpositional flap are closed with 6-0 mild chromic sutures (Plate 3-15, *B*).

An elevation of the lateral canthus can also be corrected by an adaptation of this technique. The procedure is a mirror image of the one just described; a flap of skin from the lower lid is transposed to fill a defect in the upper lid (Plate 3-15, *C* and *D*). The level of the repositioned lateral canthus is set by sighting horizontally across the patient's face and using the other three canthi as a guide to estimate the optimal location. The lateral canthal tendon is then attached to the area of Whitnall's tubercle at the lateral orbital rim with a double-armed 5-0 prolene suture with an OPS-5 needle.

Mild lower lid laxity or malposition can also be repaired with a lateral canthal tendon plication. This procedure is technically difficult and should be attempted only by someone who is very experienced with repair of lid malposition. A subciliary incision is made along the lateral eyelid and carried temporally into a smile fold 3 to 5 mm past the lateral canthal angle. Sharp dissection exposes the periosteum of the lateral canthal rim. Hemostasis is achieved with pressure and thermal cautery. The most lateral portion of the lower lid tarsus is exposed and dissected free. Both needles of a double-armed 5-0 prolene suture are passed sequentially through the lateral portion of the tarsus, from posterior to anterior. Then both needles are passed sequentially through the periosteum inside of the lateral orbital rim to suspend the lower lid and lateral canthus. The tension is adjusted to correct the lid position and laxity without causing standoff of the lateral aspect of the lower lid. The skin edges are closed with interrupted 6-0 mild chromic suture.

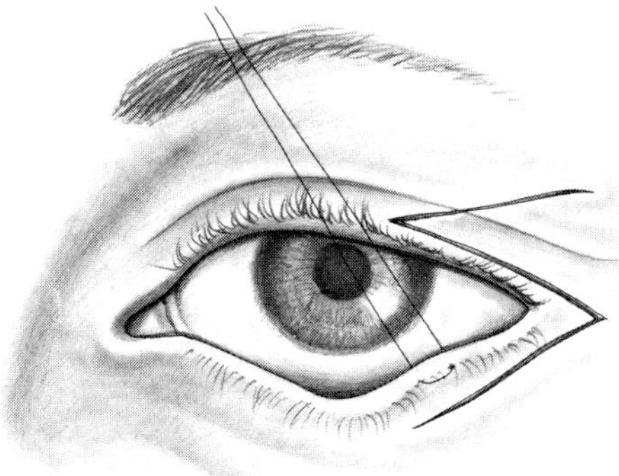
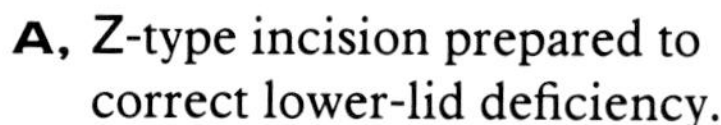

A, Z-type incision prepared to correct lower-lid deficiency.

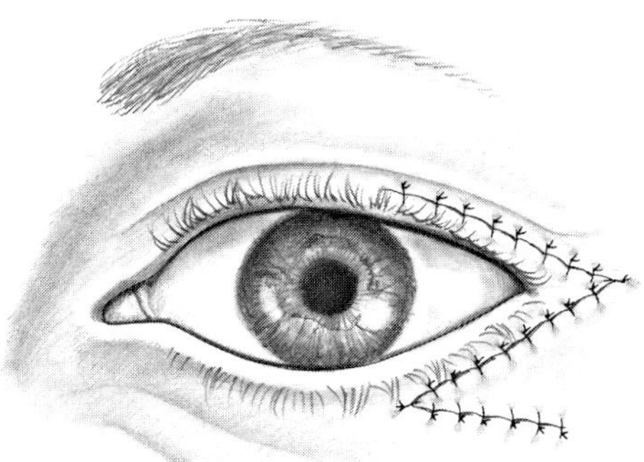

B, Upper-lid flap transposed to fill deficiency and sutured into place.

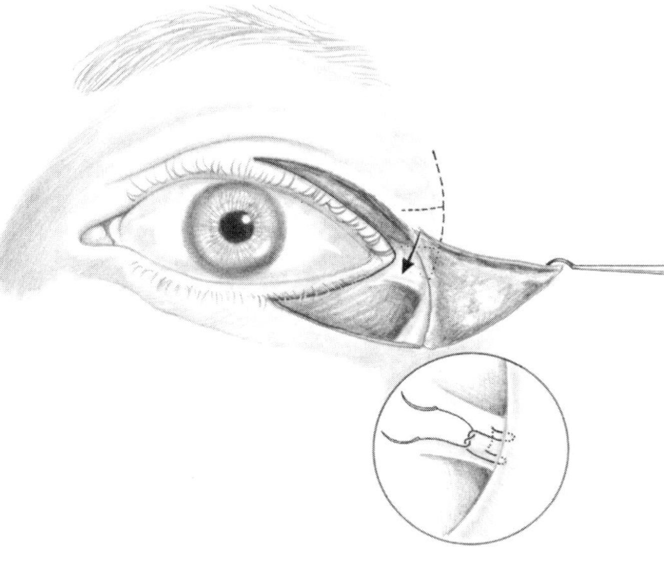

C, Central incision made along lid margin, lower flap dissected, and lateral canthal tendon repositioned.

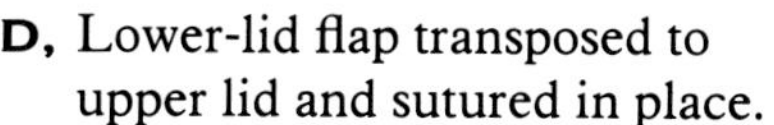

D, Lower-lid flap transposed to upper lid and sutured in place.

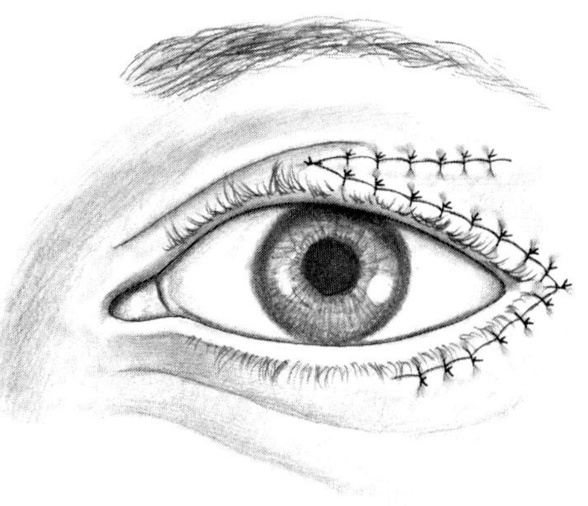

A contracted brow is a common occurrence following difficult-to-manage lacerations, chemical injuries, or thermal injuries. Z-plasty can also be used to correct these types of cicatricial brow malpositions. The new position of the elevated brow is determined by its placement in the temporal end of the lower arm of the Z. The best position can be estimated by using both the contralateral brow and the medial end of the elevated brow as landmarks. If the cilia are absent at the time of surgery, great caution should be used in the placement of the transposed flap to avoid splitting the brow cilia.

The central incision in this case is placed under and parallel to the brow cilia. The incision is beveled 30 degrees with respect to brow cilia and their roots, which are angled 30 degrees to the skin surface. The superior arm of the incision is then offset to follow the superior orbital rim (Plate 3-16, *A*). The flaps are dissected. Damage to the cilia is minimized by gentle, precise dissection and appropriate beveling of the incision. However, the cilia may still temporarily fall out. The flaps are transposed, with the temporal end of the lower incision receiving the extremity of the elevated brow (Plate 3-16, *B*). The flaps are sutured in place with interrupted 6-0 mild sutures. A light pressure patch is applied for the first postoperative day.

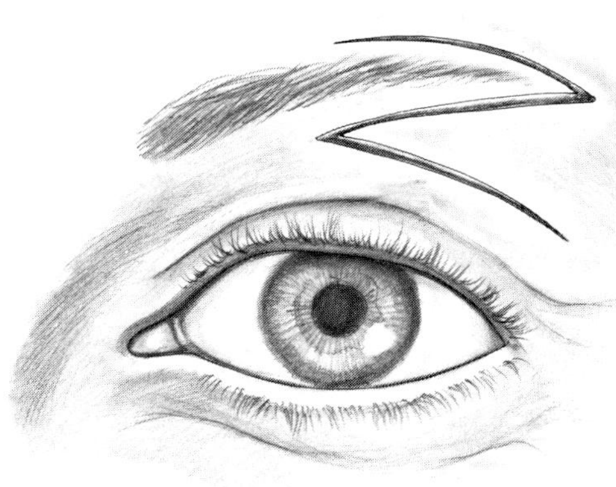

A, Correction of elevated brow by Z-type incision.

B, Transposed brow, with placement at temporal end of lower arm.

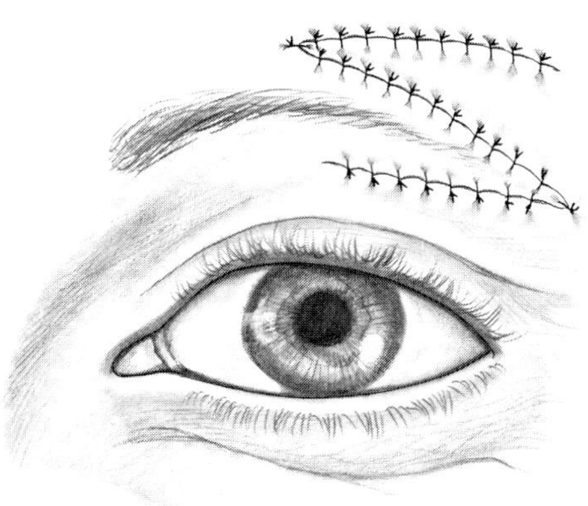

GRAFTING TECHNIQUES

Free skin grafts and tarsal grafts are especially useful techniques among the many options available to the ophthalmic reconstructive surgeon. A knowledge of the basic procedures used in free skin grafting and their more common clinical applications will enable the surgeon to apply the procedures to almost any case in which skin grafting is required. Tarsal grafts are used to reinforce or augment the internal lamellae of the lids. They may be used alone or in combination with free skin grafts, but two nonvascularized grafts should not be sutured together.

The skin is divided into the epidermal layer and the dermal layer. The subdermal fat is just below the dermal layer. A split-thickness skin graft refers to any graft that is less than the full thickness of the skin. A full-thickness skin graft utilizes all of the skin layers and frequently has a small amount of the subdermal fat attached to it (Plate 4-1). Full-thickness skin grafts give the best color and texture match when they are taken from the contralateral lid. The next best match is skin obtained from any lid. Lid skin is frequently not available for grafting in reconstruction cases. In these cases, retroauricular skin makes an excellent substitute and is usually in adequate supply and acceptable condition. If these areas are not available for skin graft harvesting, supraclavicular skin can be used. Split-thickness skin grafts may also be used. Full-thickness skin grafts are usually obtained freehand, and split-thickness skin grafts are usually obtained with a dermatome.

A certain amount of postoperative graft contracture is expected. A full-thickness graft will shrink approximately 25% of its original size. A split-thickness graft will shrink approximately 50% of its original size. The clinical significance of this contracture is minimized by oversizing the grafts an appropriate amount and by placing the graft site on stretch for the first postoperative week. Occasionally, dermabrasion is useful to modify the graft if its appearance is not acceptable after several months of observation.

Dermal, fat, and dermis-fat grafts are useful for volume replacement. They are obtained by removing a measured block of tissue from a suitable site, usually the lateral buttocks, and dissecting off the overlying epidermis and dermis, as required. These layers may be removed with dermabrasion or a dermatome. We prefer to inject the dermis with local anesthetic and remove the epidermis freehand.

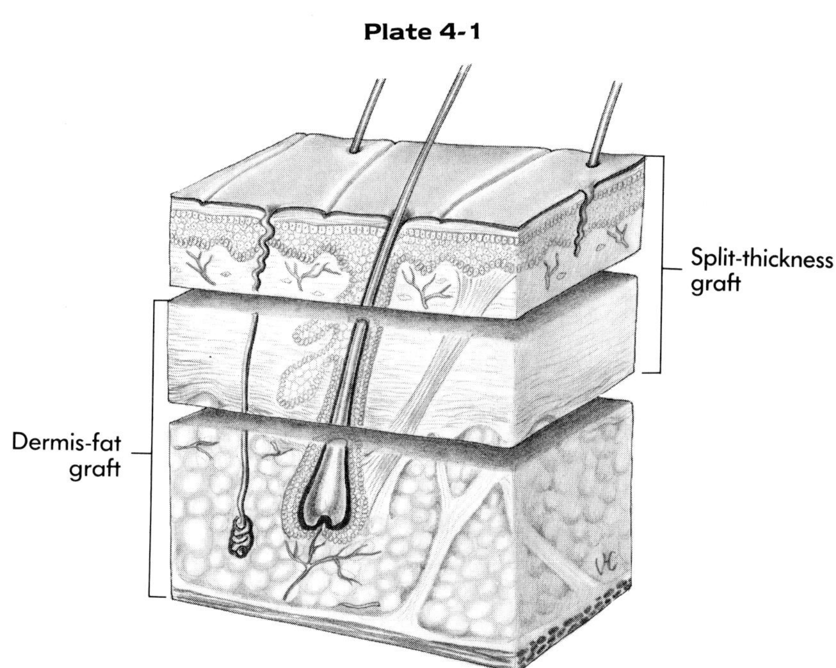

Layers of the skin: epidermis, dermis, fat.

Extensive trauma to the upper lid may cause a contracted scar and a decrease in the vertical dimension of the lid, for which a Z-plasty is insufficient. In such cases, a free skin graft may be needed to replace the scar tissue that is excised and thus to release the retracted lid. A 4-0 silk suture is passed through the lid margin, and an elliptical incision is made in the upper lid. The lower border of the incision is parallel to the lid margin. The upper border forms an arc. The two incisions enclose all of the cicatricial tissue between them (Plate 4-2, *A*).

The surgeon excises the contracted tissue with sharp dissection. Any underlying fibrotic bands are incised and removed. The traction suture is used to continually test the remaining tension within the lid during the excision of the cicatricial tissue. Once the lid has been sufficiently released, the 4-0 silk suture is anchored to the area overlying the inferior orbital rim (Plate 4-2, *B*), with the upper lid actually overriding the lower lid. Hemostasis of the recipient site is best achieved by including epinephrine in the local anesthetic and by applying gentle pressure to the site with a moist gauze and/or a charged collagen hemostatic compound, such as Helistat. Excessive use of cautery may cause the graft to be lost because of insufficient blood supply.

The donor site is selected on the basis of the size of the graft required and the sites available. The size of the graft is marked on a piece of Telfa by pressing it against the recipient bed, which will stain the Telfa with a light layer of blood. The Telfa is then cut into an appropriately oversized template and placed on the donor site. The graft is marked out. It is ballooned away from deeper tissue with an injection of 1% lidocaine with 1:100,000 epinephrine into the subcutaneous tissues. Full-thickness skin is excised while being handled very gently (Plate 4-2, *C*). It is kept over the patient's sterile drape at all times. A small amount of underlying subcutaneous tissue will always come with the graft. This excess tissue is removed by placing the graft, epidermis side down, against a gloved, nondominant index finger and using scissors to trim off all of the fatty-appearing tissue. It is better to leave a small amount of subcutaneous tissue than to repeatedly cut through the skin graft.

The graft is immediately transferred to the recipient bed and sutured into place with interrupted 6-0 mild chromic sutures (Plate 4-2, *D*). The graft is incised with a razor knife at several places, like a pie crust, to prevent fluid accumulation under it. A layer of antibiotic ointment is placed on the graft before a bolster is placed over the graft. The ointment is helpful to keep the graft soft and to allow easier removal of the bolster. The bolster is made of a bottom layer of moist Telfa, to prevent adhesion between the graft and the bolster, and an upper layer of rolled, moist cotton to provide rigidity. It is anchored with interrupted 6-0 mild chromic sutures placed several millimeters away from the edge of the graft. This prevents traction on the graft margin and reduces the effort necessary to find all of the small residual pieces of suture when the bolster is removed in the office. An additional layer of antibiotic ointment is placed on the bolster, and a pressure patch is placed over the bolster. The pressure patch is removed by the patient the following day.

The donor site is closed last. Cautery may be used as required. A donor site requiring minimal tension to join the skin edges is closed with interrupted 6-0 mild chromic sutures. A donor site requiring moderate or greater tension is closed with interrupted 4-0 black nylon suture to allow adequate wound healing time.

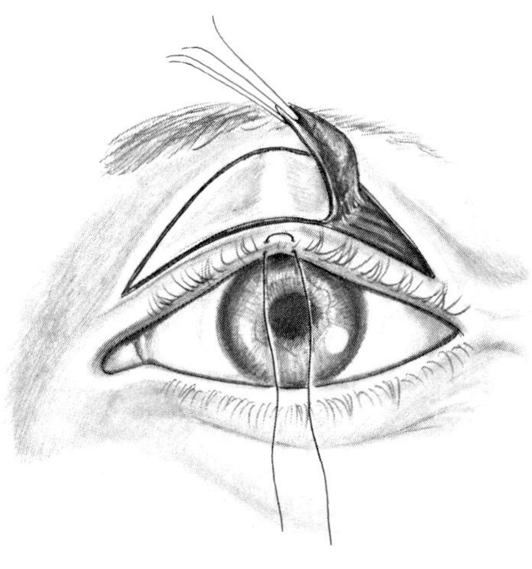

A. Excision of scar with 4-0 silk traction suture in place.

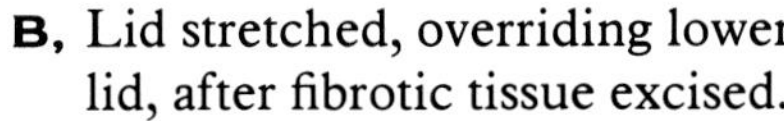

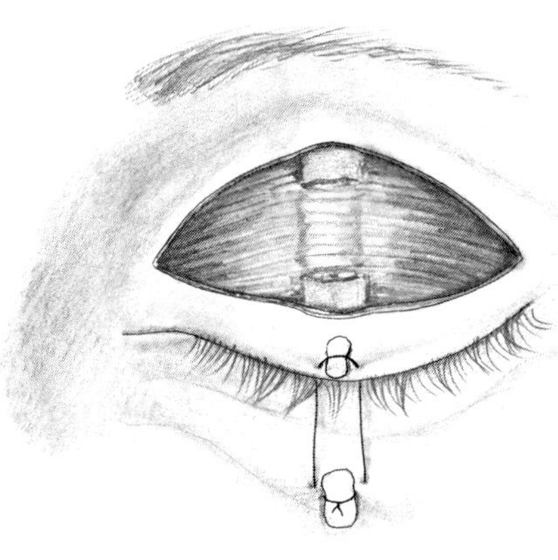

B. Lid stretched, overriding lower lid, after fibrotic tissue excised.

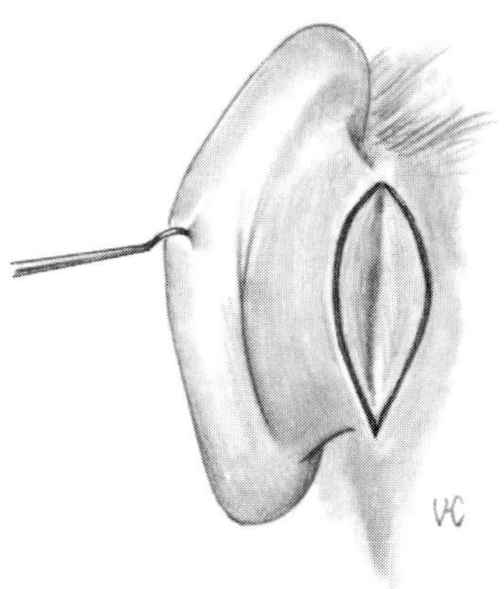

C. Full-thickness skin is harvested from the retroauricular area.

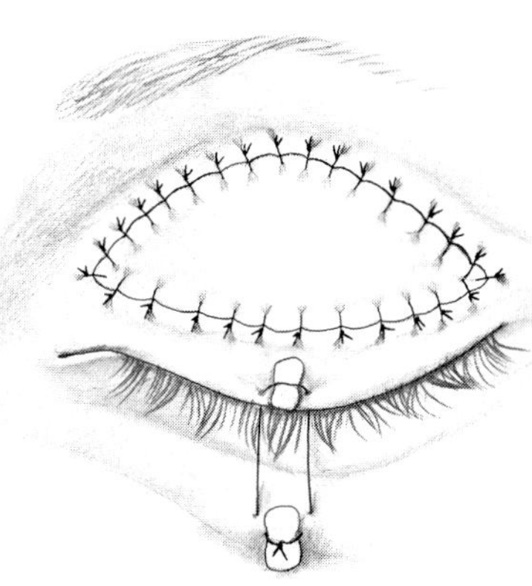

D. Full-thickness skin graft sutured in place.

Injury to the internal lamellae of the lower lids can cause retraction and subsequent vertical shortening (Plate 4-3, *A*). Retraction of the lower lid to a level below the inferior limbus after trauma, associated with an increased stiffness of the lid, suggests scarring of the internal lamella of the lid. A free auricular cartilage graft is often required to reconstruct lids with this type of scarring.

A 4-0 silk traction suture is placed in the lower eyelid, and the eyelid is everted over a retractor (Plate 4-3, *B*). An incision is made through the palpebral conjunctiva and capsulopalpebral fascia at the inferior border of the tarsal plate. The incision is extended several millimeters nasally and temporally past the ends of the tarsal plate. It detaches the capsulopalpebral fascia and the lower eyelid retractors. Hemostasis is achieved with thermal cautery, and attention is directed toward the donor site.

The outer edge of the ear is anesthetized. The lid is incised just anterior to the outer edge of the ear. An incision is made along this mark for 25 to 30 mm. The incision is only through skin and subcutaneous tissues. Curved iris scissors are used to expose the ear cartilage anteriorly. A razor knife is used to dissect the graft (Plate 4-3, *C*). The width of the graft is the height the lower lid needs to be elevated. The length of the graft is the length of the lower lid tarsus, usually about 30 mm. Cautery and direct pressure on the ear will control the bleeding. The skin is closed at the end of the procedure with interrupted 6-0 mild chromic sutures from skin to skin only. Attention is directed to the lower eyelid.

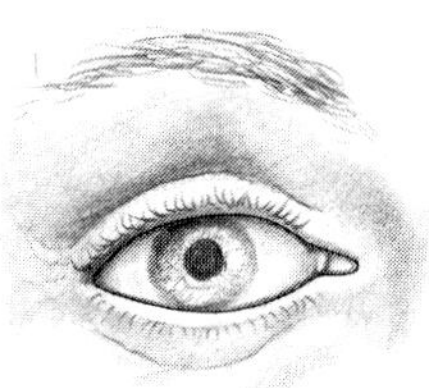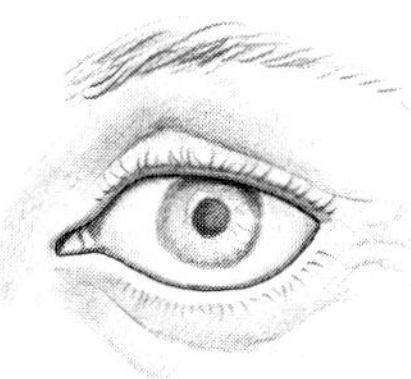

A, Vertically shortened left lower lid.

B, Infratarsal incision indicated from nasal to temporal extremity.

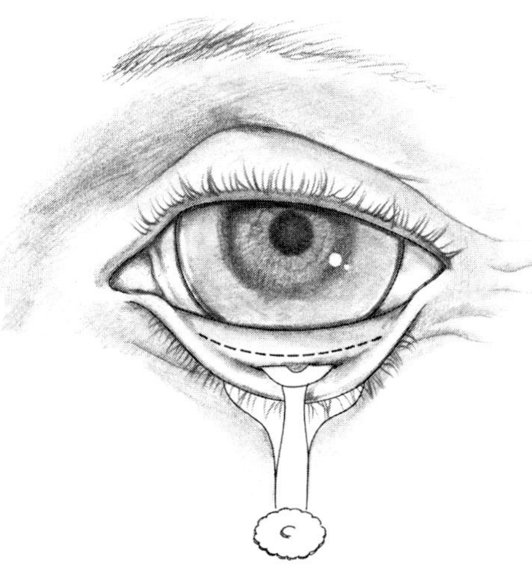

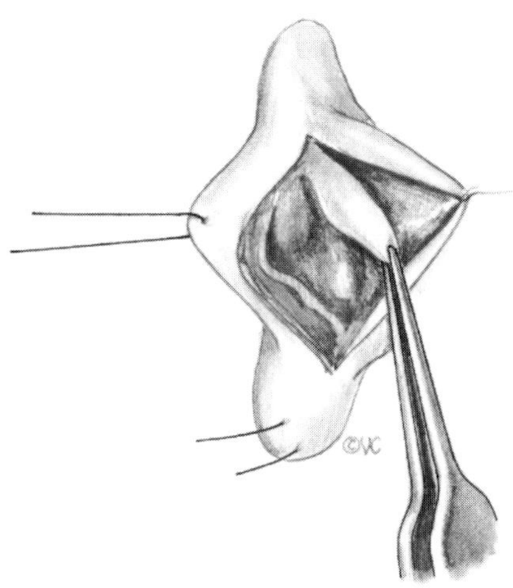

C, Ear cartilage is harvested.

The ear cartilage is trimmed and brought into position just below the tarsal plate. It is anchored in position with interrupted, inverted 5-0 Vicryl sutures (Plate 4-3, *D*). The knots must be below the internal surface of the lid to avoid excessive ocular irritation. A surgical assistant is very helpful throughout this procedure, but is especially vital during initial anchoring of the graft. Approximately 6 sutures on the upper border and 6 sutures on the lower border of the graft are required. The ends of the graft are sutured last, after final trimming of the graft has been accomplished. The 4-0 silk suture is taped to the brow (Plate 4-3, *E*) and removed after 4 to 5 days. The ear cartilage acts as a spacer between the inferior border of the tarsus and the lower eyelid retractors. The cross-sectional view reveals the ear cartilage graft sutured into position, with correction of the lower eyelid contraction. The patient will experience some irritation until the surface of the graft becomes epithelialized in 2 to 6 weeks.

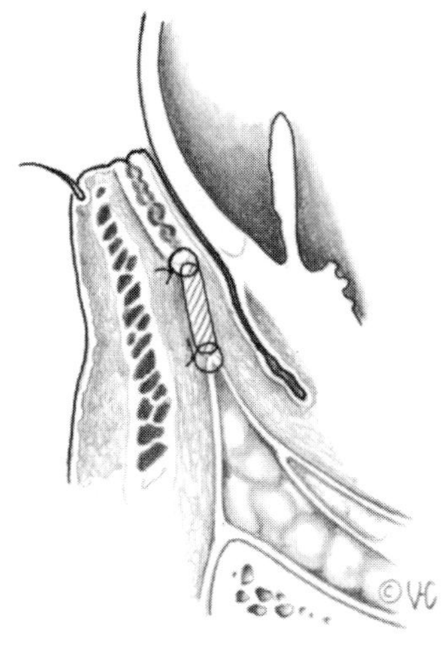

D, Ear cartilage graft sutured into position.

E, 4-0 silk suture taped to brow.

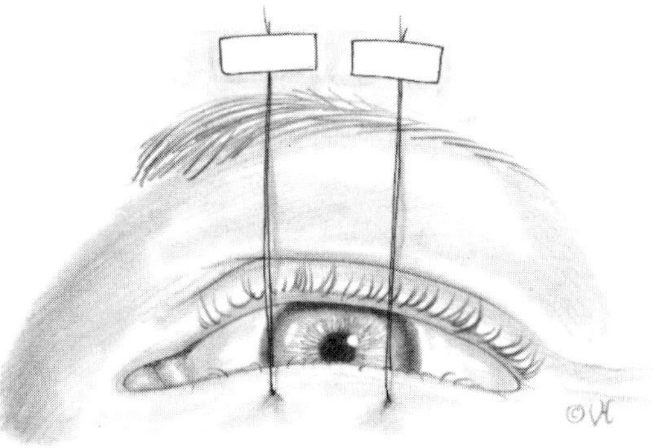

CHAPTER 5

LID TRAUMA

The repair of soft-tissue injury to the eyelids involves the use of refined surgical and microsurgical techniques, as well as the technical advances that have been made in instrumentation and suture manufacture.

The initial examination includes evaluating the patient for the possibility of direct or indirect ocular injury. A slit-lamp examination of the anterior segment and anterior vitreous and a funduscopic examination are prerequisites to evaluation and repair of the adnexal trauma. The possibility of neurologic deficits in cases of severe trauma must be considered, with neurologic and neurosurgical consultation as needed.

After the neurologic status and ocular status of the patient have been stabilized, attention is turned to the periorbital tissue. The area should be cleansed of debris and blood. Evidence of tissue loss should be sought, because the missing tissue can often be located. Following an appropriate preoperative evaluation, surgical repair is begun.

Full-thickness lacerations of the lid margin should be repaired with the classic three-suture technique, provided there is no significant tissue loss and the wound edges are clean and regular. Any irregular wound margins and those with tissue loss are best closed by creating a pentagonal wedge resection of the wound margins (Plate 5-1, *A* and *B*). This will allow better apposition of the lid margin and will minimize any tendency to form secondary cicatricial ectropion or entropion. A protective shell may be placed over the globe, but will tend to distort the lid being repaired. Anesthesia is achieved with infiltration of 1% lidocaine with 1:100,000 epinephrine. This solution is infiltrated even when general anesthesia is utilized, to control intraoperative bleeding.

Double-armed 6-0 silk suture is passed from the lacerated edge through the meibomian orifices of lid margin, 1 to 2 mm from the wound margin. The depth of the pass should approximate the distance from the wound edge. The other end of the 6-0 silk suture is passed into the lacerated margin and out of the meibomian orifices in a mirror-like fashion. The suture ends are now crossed and the margin brought together. The margin should be in good position, and the edges should be well-apposed. If the lid margin is not fully corrected at this point, the silk suture should be withdrawn and passed again. After the first suture has established the correct relationship between both halves of the lid laceration, it is secured with three throws and the needles are removed from the sutures.

The second silk suture is placed posterior to the first suture, at the mucocutaneous junction. The third suture is placed anterior to the first suture, at the lash line; care is taken not to place the suture anterior to the lash line, to avoid inward rotation of the lid margin. Both sutures are tied with three throws. Their tails are left long, and their needles are removed. At this stage, the lid margin should be smooth and continuous except for a slight puckering of lid margin between the silk sutures. The tarsal plate is re-approximated with 5-0 Vicryl sutures through its anterior surface and lacerated edge (Plate 5-1, *C*). Generally, two Vicryl sutures are required for the upper lid and a single Vicryl for the lower lid. The remainder of the laceration is closed with interrupted 6-0 mild chromic sutures. The tails of the silk sutures are now brought anterior and tied away from the eye, with a final 6-0 silk suture through the skin only several millimeters away from the lash line. The last suture is trimmed close to the knot, along with the tails of the three primary silk sutures (Plate 5-1, *D*).

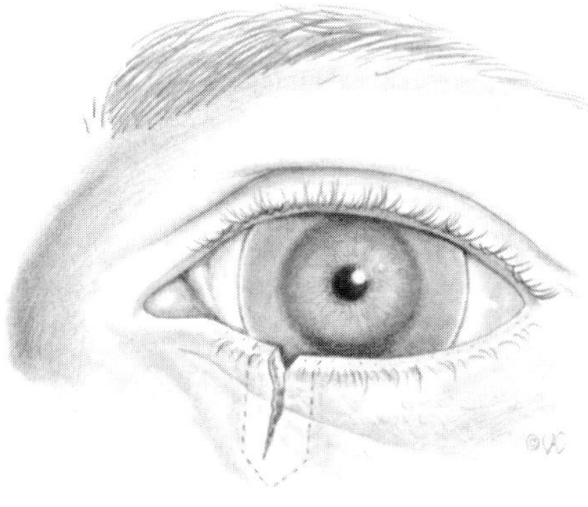

A, Irregular wound margins are marked in pentagonal fashion.

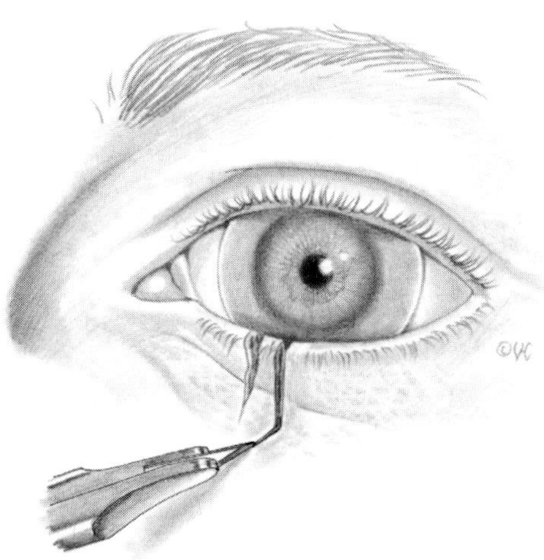

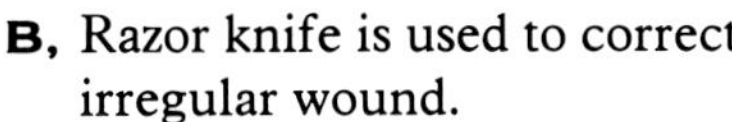

B, Razor knife is used to correct irregular wound.

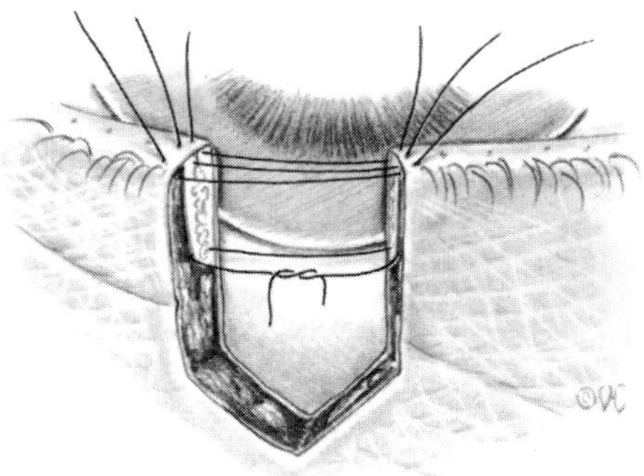

C, 6-0 silk sutures used to close lid margin and 5-0 Vicryl to close tarsus.

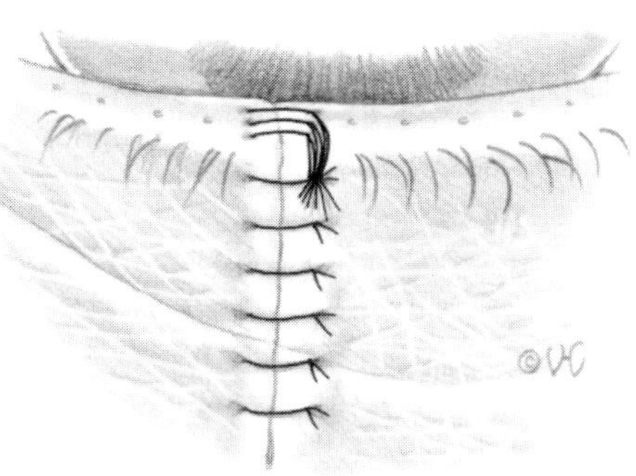

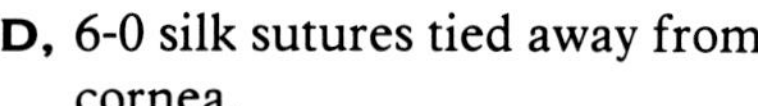

D, 6-0 silk sutures tied away from cornea.

The intregrity of the lacrimal drainage system must be reestablished after transmarginal lacerations involving the canaliculi in the area between the punctum and the medial canthus (Plate 5-2). Although most patients with a single functioning canaliculus remain asymptomatic, some can have significant epiphora. Therefore, a laceration of a single canaliculus should usually be repaired. A possible exception to this rule is a laceration of a single canaliculus in a patient likely to have decreased tear production. Another good argument for not repairing the canalicular rupture primarily is relative inexperience of the surgeon at repairing lacrimal system trauma. A traumatic intubation of the uninvolved canaliculus could damage both canaliculi and, potentially, could necessitate a conjunctivodacryocystorhinostomy to repair the damage.

A transmarginal lid laceration is often associated with lacrimal system ruptures. Recent evidence suggests indirect trauma is a more common cause of canalicular ruptures than direct trauma. Any canalicular laceration should prompt a thorough evaluation of the lids, orbit, and globe to avoid missing any occult damage.

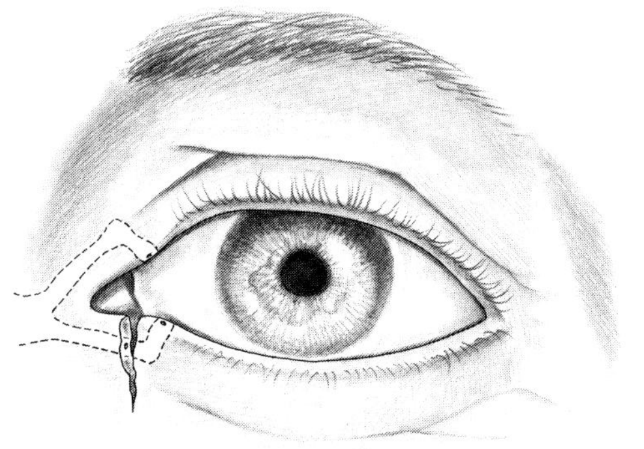

Full-thickness lid laceration
involving lower canaliculus.

Both canaliculi should be examined on the operating table for inapparent damage and debris. If only a single canaliculus is involved, it should be intubated before the uninvolved canaliculus (Plate 5-3, *A*). If it cannot be intubated, the laceration should be closed with repair of the lacrimal system rather than place the entire system at risk. Injection of dye into the uninvolved system to facilitate identification of the distal portion of the ruptured canaliculus is acceptable, but both ends of the canaliculus can usually be identified by direct visualization or, if necessary, with the aid of the operating microscope.

Use of Silastic tubing, with a malleable tip at each end, is the preferred method of canalicular intubation. The malleable tips are retrieved from the nose with a hook or guide. Some practice is usually necessary to make retrieval of the tips possible.

Severed tendon structures and subcutaneous tissue are closed with 5-0 absorbable suture; sutures are placed to decrease tension on the wound (Plate 5-3, *B*). Proper closure of the severed canaliculus is then mandatory; 9-0 or 10-0 Ethilon suture or 8-0 Vicryl suture is used to meticulously close the canaliculus (Plate 5-3, *C*). With the tension-relieving suture in place, cheese wiring of the canaliculus can be avoided.

The lid margin is then closed with 6-0 silk suture, with the usual technique. The Silastic tubing is tied in the nose with a simple knot (Plate 5-3, *D*).

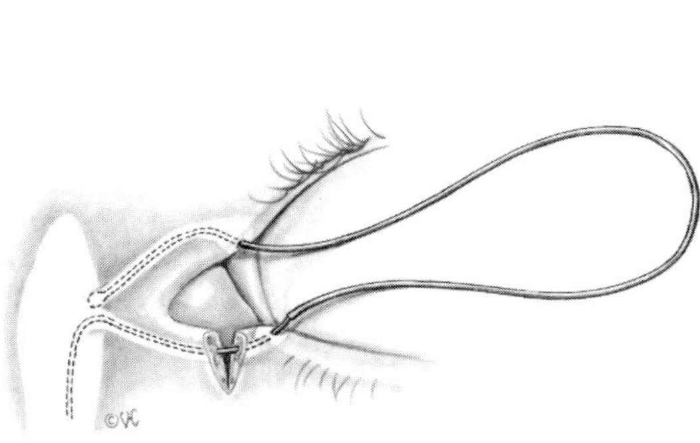

A, Severed canaliculus is intubated before uninvolved one.

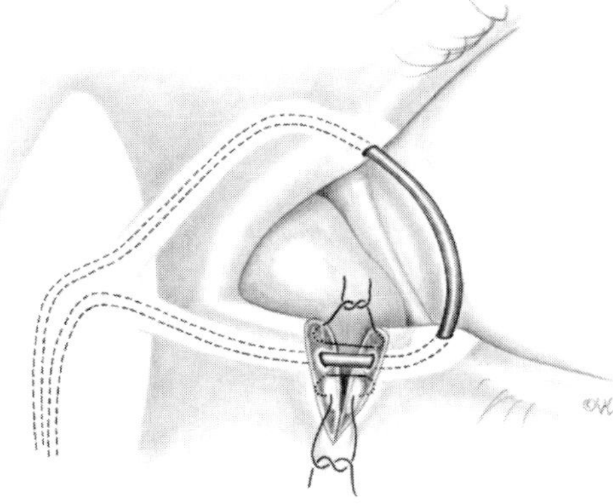

B, Severed canthal tendon and subcutaneous structures are closed with 5-0 absorbable suture.

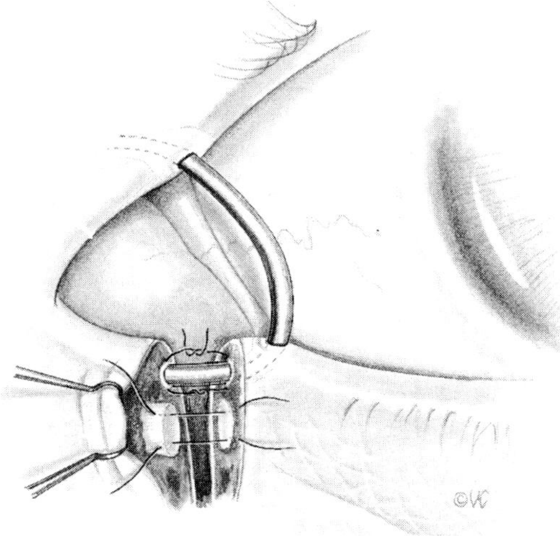

C, 9-0 or 10-0 ethilon (or 8-0 Vicryl) suture is used to repair the severed canaliculus.

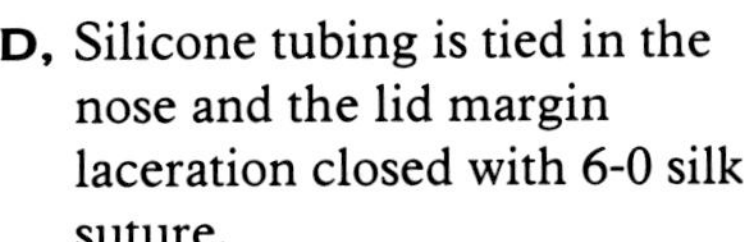

D, Silicone tubing is tied in the nose and the lid margin laceration closed with 6-0 silk suture.

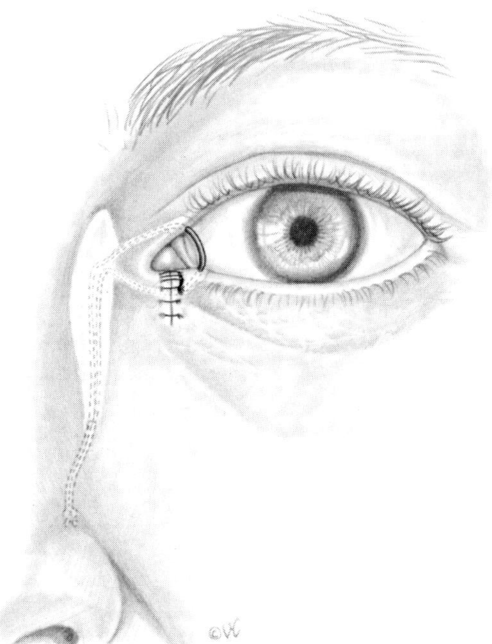

The superficial heads of the pretarsal muscle unite to form the medial canthal tendon. Often in transmarginal lacerations involving the canaliculus, the superficial heads forming the canthal tendon are severed and difficult to locate (Plate 5-4, *A*).

A simple method of locating these structures is to make a vertical incision over the insertion of the medial canthal tendon and dissect down to its periosteal insertion (Plate 5-4, *B*). To minimize bleeding, it is helpful to inject the area with 1% lidocaine with 1:100,000 epinephrine 20 minutes prior to making the incision.

Blunt scissors are used to trace the course of the superficial heads of the pretarsal orbicularis back to the point at which they are severed. These are anastomosed directly with 5-0 prolene (Plate 5-4, *C*). (This incision is also indicated in injuries directly involving the medial canthal tendon.) The canaliculi and transmarginal laceration are then closed as previously described. The incision over the medial canthal tendon is closed with interrupted 6-0 mild chromic sutures (Plate 5-4, *D*).

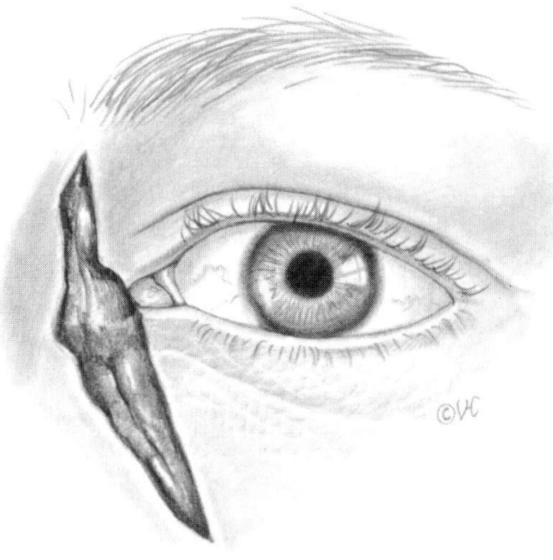

A, Laceration involving canaliculus and medial canthal tendon.

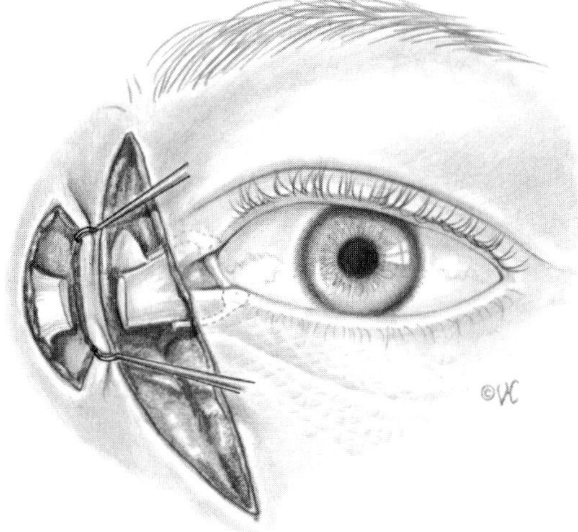

B, Vertical incision made over insertion of medial canthal tendon.

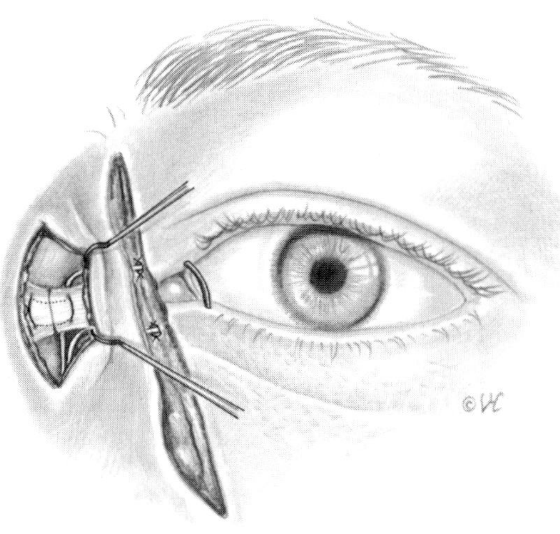

C, 5-0 prolene suture used to re-approximate the medial canthal tendon.

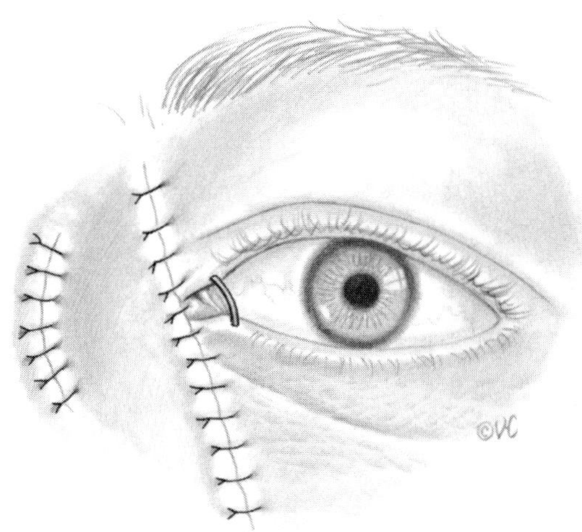

D, Overlying lacerations are then closed.

CHAPTER 6

EXCISION OF MARGINAL LID TUMORS

The variability in the presentation of malignant marginal lid tumors often makes the diagnosis a difficult one, and therefore any lesion of the lid margin that leaves even a modicum of doubt in the surgeon's mind should be sent for microscopic diagnosis.

EXCISIONAL BIOPSY

Although the history of the evolution of a lid mass can be useful to the surgeon and even though serial photography can be used to follow its progression, we generally prefer the simple certainty of an excisional biopsy of these tumors to ensure peace of mind, to the patient and the surgeon.

Raised lesion (Plate 6-1)

The type of excisional biopsy depends on the shape, size, and location of the lesion. For raised lesions of the lid margin, we generally prefer a shave excision. The eyelid below the mass is anesthetized with 1% lidocaine with 1:100,000 epinephrine, and the blood vessels are allowed to constrict for several minutes. The lid is pulled away from the globe, and the surgeon places a stiff, flat instrument between the globe and the eyelid (Plate 6-1). A scalpel is used to shave off all of the mass that is greater than a half-millimeter above the lid margin. A hand-held thermal cautery is used to obtain hemostasis and to bevel the lid margin to its normal contour. A patch is not necessary, but a small amount of antibiotic ointment will keep the scar soft and free of infection.

Inferiorly directed lesion (Plate 6-2)

For inferiorly directed lesions the blade of the knife is turned in the opposite direction (Plate 6-2), and with the same sawing motion, this time away from the globe, the lesion is excised, with care to leave the lash roots intact, in the event that the lesion is benign. Thermal cautery is again used to sculpt the incision.

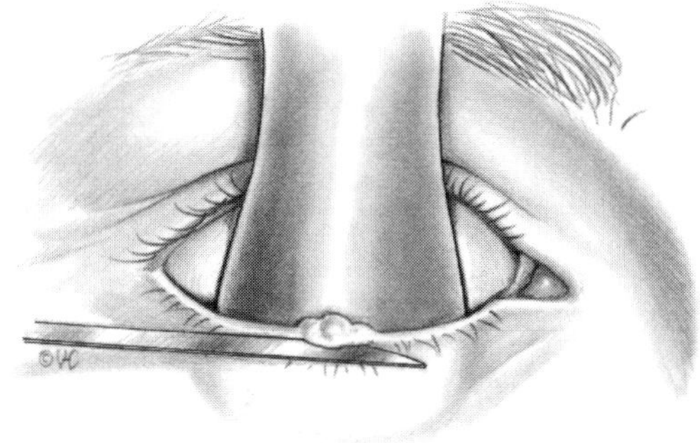

Knife blade used to excise a raised lesion.

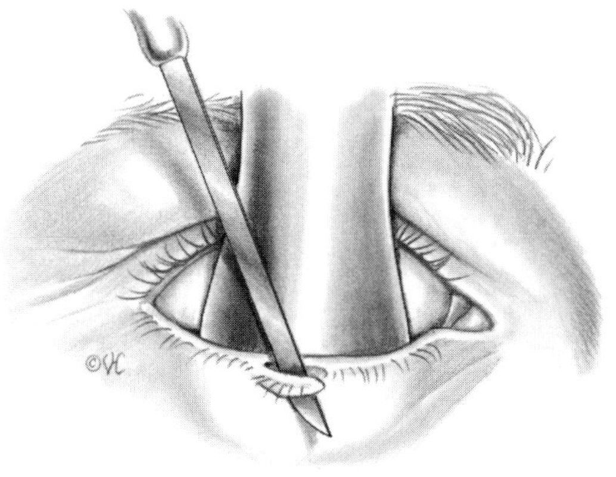

Lash roots left in place as inferiorly directed lesion is excised.

A flat lesion of the eyelid margin is removed in a fashion similar to that for an elevated lesion. The lid is anesthetized and allowed to sit for several minutes. The lid is pulled away from the globe, and a globe protector is inserted into the lower fornix. A scalpel tip is pushed into the lateral extent of the mass, and the incision is extended through the medial margin of the mass (Plate 6-3, *A* and *B*). The medial margin of the mass is grasped, and the incision is extended laterally to complete the excision of the mass (Plate 6-3, *C* and *D*). Thermal cautery is used to achieve hemostasis and to bevel the lid margin to its normal contour.

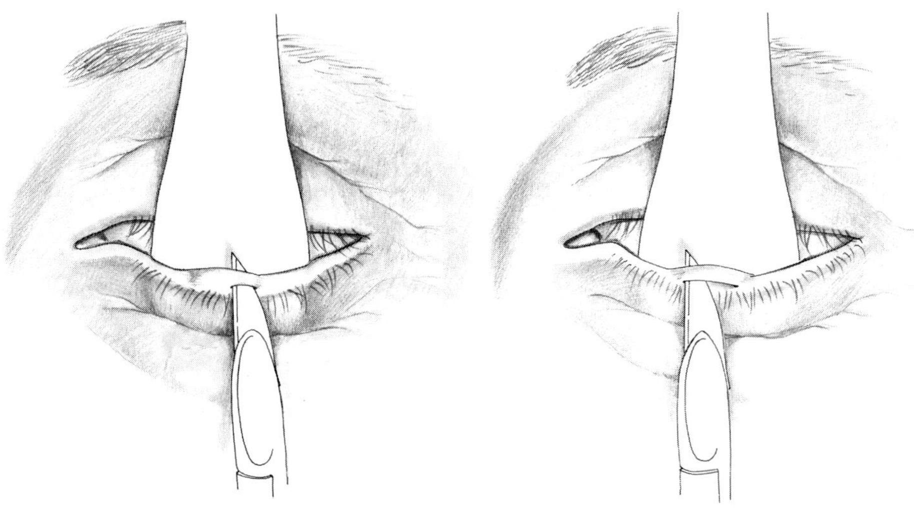

A, Razor knife perforates flat lesion at lateral extremity.

B, Lesion incised to medial extremity.

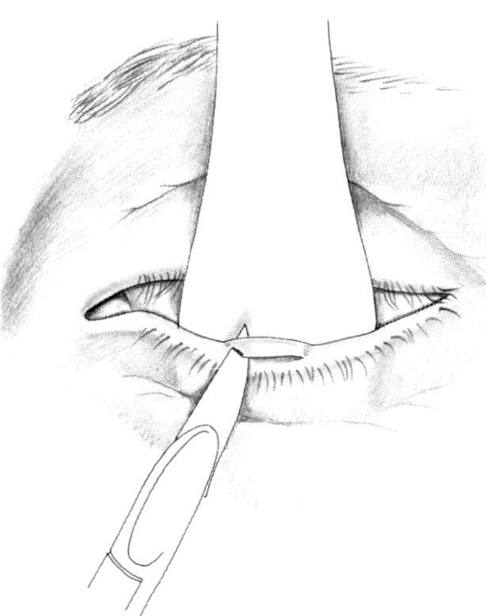

C, Medial edge of lesion cut free.

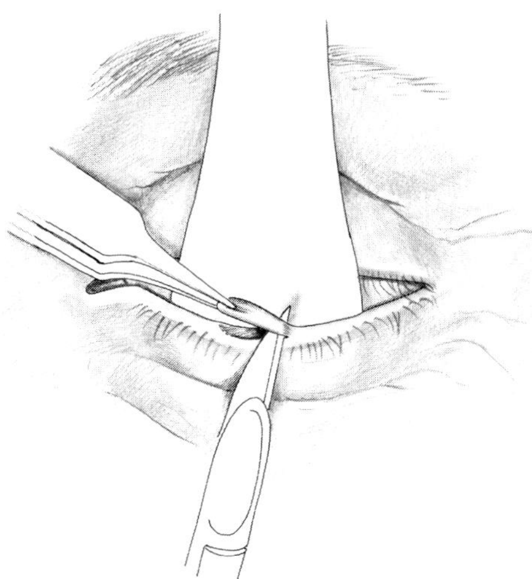

D, Excision of lesion being completed.

Dermabrasion is a useful technique for the removal of small benign lesions or scars of the lid margin. The area is infiltrated with an equal mixture of 1% lidocaine and 0.75% Marcaine, both with 1:100,000 epinephrine. The area is firmly abraded with a piece of sandpaper wrapped around the dominant index finger while a lid plate is used to protect the globe (Plate 6-4, *A* and *B*). The endpoint is a slow, uniform oozing from the dermabraded area. A mechanical dermabrader can be hand held and used in a similar fashion (Plate 6-4, *C*). Mechanically assisted dermabrasion should not be attempted on the eyelids by anyone except the most experienced surgeon. It is too easy to cut completely through the skin and into the subcutaneous tissues. We rarely use mechanically assisted dermabrasion. Patients frequently require strong pain medications for several days after dermabrasion.

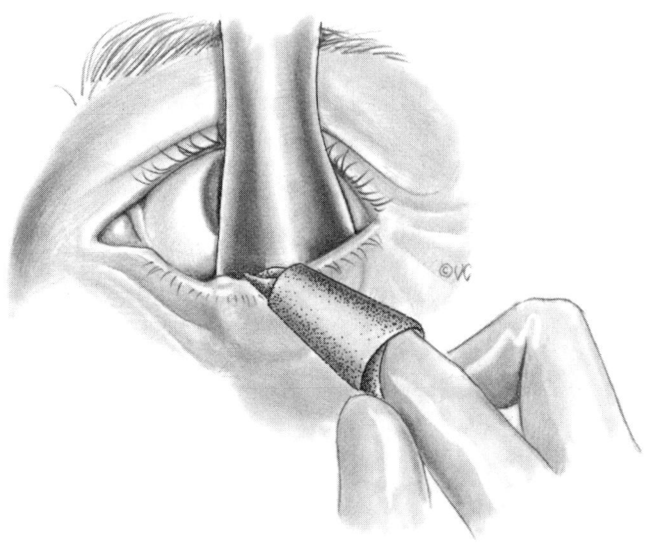

A, Fine sandpaper used to level tumor mass.

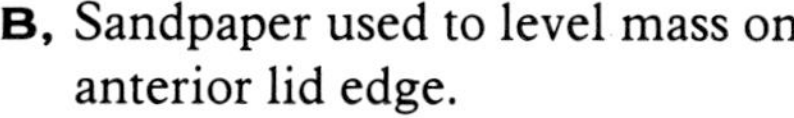

B, Sandpaper used to level mass on anterior lid edge.

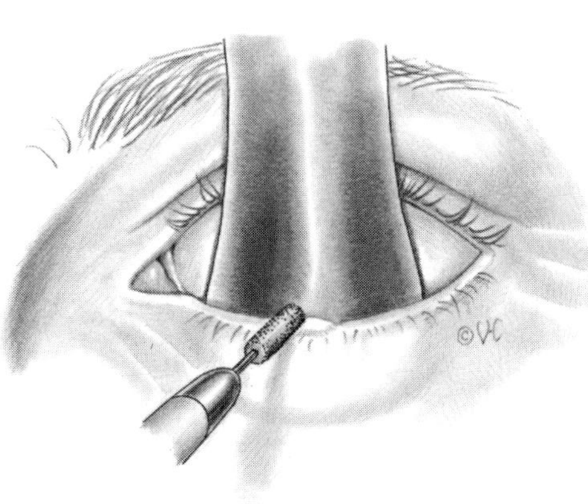

C, Mechanical dermabrader used to level lid mass.

An en bloc resection with microscopic control of surgical margins is required for malignant eyelid lesions (Plate 6-5, *A* and *B*). We prefer surgical techniques that will ensure complete extirpation of the tumor mass, giving thought to reconstruction of the eyelid only after the tumor has been completely excised. One of the major causes of recurrent malignant tumors is failure to completely excise the lesion during the primary surgery, because of the patient's and the surgeon's apprehension at the thought of a major reconstructive procedure.

The limits of the lesion should be estimated preoperatively, but the surgeon must remember that it is not possible to reliably estimate the extent of the lesion clinically. In the presence of a malignancy, the meibomian gland orifices are usually obliterated or deranged. It is usually necessary to go beyond the abnormal architecture by two or three meibomian orifices to be likely to enclose the tumor in the excision (Plate 6-5, *C*).

After the en bloc specimen is excised and sent for permanent section processing, 1-mm-thick strips of tissue from the entire raw margin are removed, labeled, and sent for frozen sections. Processing the specimens in this fashion minimizes the potential for miscommunication between the surgeon and the pathologist. Any malignancy seen in the strips sent for frozen sections represents a positive margin and necessitates further excision. The pentagonal wedge is closed with the classic three-suture technique (Plate 6-5, *D* and *E*).

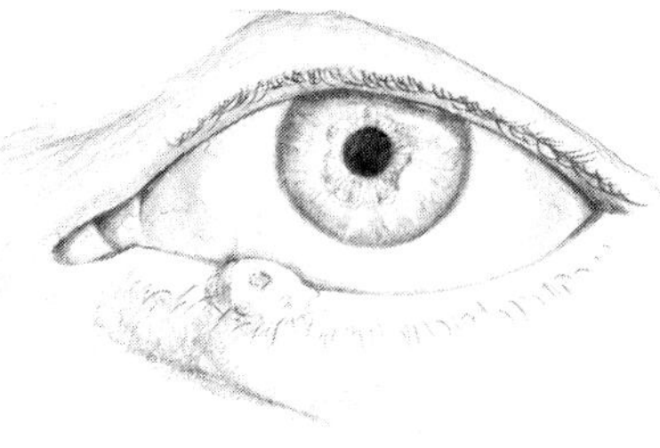

A, Malignant lesion occupying medial one third of lower lid.

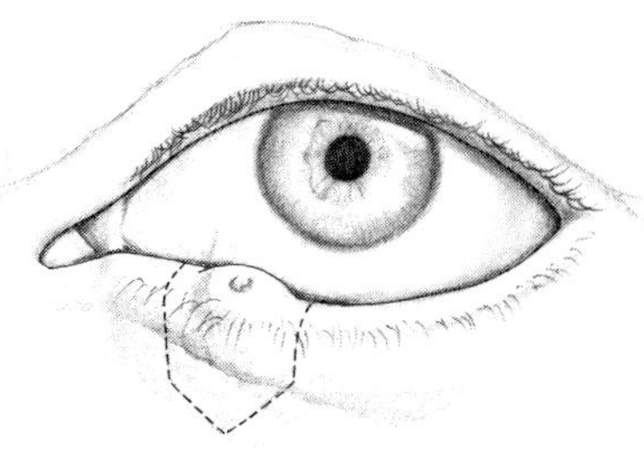

B, Margin of excision extends two to three normal meibomian orifices beyond lesion.

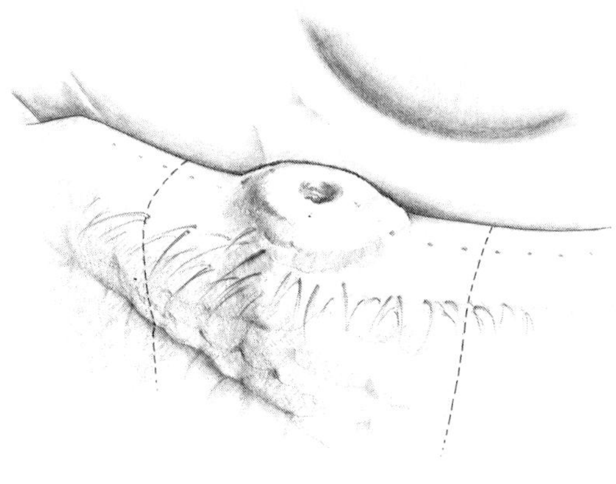

C, Area to be excised, with marginal and basal sections slated for excision.

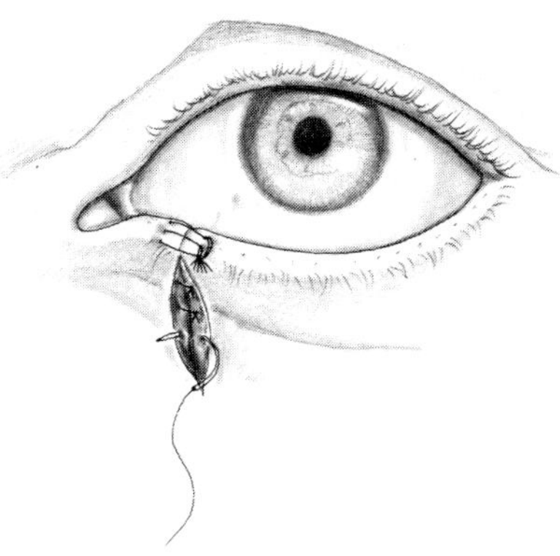

D, Closure of lid defect with three-suture technique.

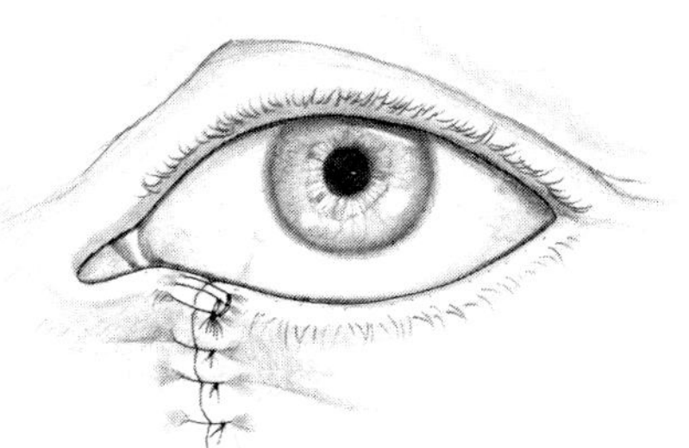

E, Lid defect suture closed.

EYELID RECONSTRUCTION

The reconstructive surgeon operating on the ocular adnexa needs to be familiar with a series of procedures that will enable him or her to successfully repair eyelid defects ranging from a simple lid laceration to replacement of large volumes of lost tissue. The surgeon's ability to perform this type of surgery is based on the knowledge of the normal regional anatomy and an understanding of the fundamental principles of ophthalmic plastic surgery. The surgeon should always have in mind a stepwise plan for solving progressively complex reconstructive problems in accordance with the size and location of the defect.

Since a primary closure cannot always be achieved, the surgeon should be prepared to employ lid-lengthening procedures such as lateral canthotomy and cantholysis and proceed to composite grafts and lateral advancement flaps when these fail. In the event that even more tissue is required for reconstruction, he or she should be familiar with the use of tarsoconjunctival flaps, bridge flaps, transposition flaps, lined pedicle flaps, and Mustardé-type techniques for lower and upper lid use. Because of the very unusual anatomy of the canthi, the procedures and principles described here are unique.

A deficiency in the horizontal dimension of the eyelid is termed a coloboma, whether it is traumatic, congenital, or iatrogenic. The type of closure is the same as that for a transmarginal laceration. However, a very large defect may require a more complex reconstructive procedure. The rounded edges of a congenital or long-standing traumatic coloboma need to be trimmed with a pentagonal wedge resection to allow precise apposition of the wound edges (Plate 7-1).

The proposed excision is delineated with a surgical marking pen (Plate 7-1, *A*). The area is infiltrated with 1% lidocaine with 1:100,000 epinephrine and allowed to vasoconstrict for several minutes. The margin of the defect is grasped while a razor knife is used to create a smooth raw edge (Plate 7-1, *B*). The lid margin is closed with the previously described three-suture technique. The tarsus is closed with 5-0 Vicryl sutures. The overlying skin is closed with interrupted 6-0 mild chromic sutures (Plate 7-1, *C*).

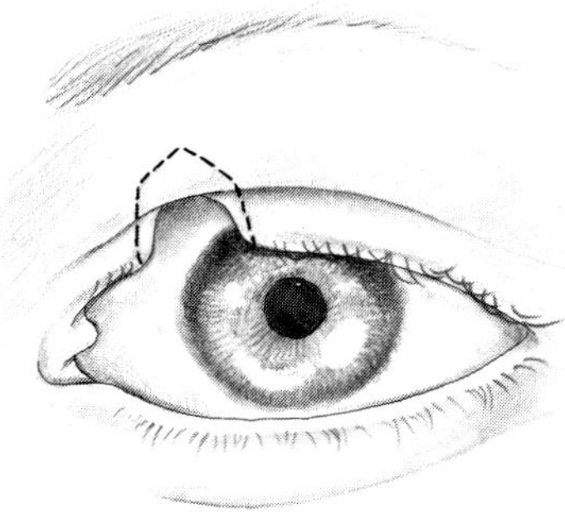

A, Coloboma of nasal aspect of upper lid.

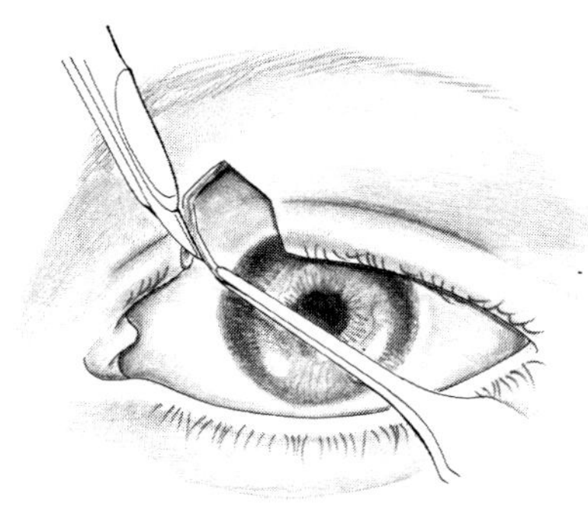

B, Marginal tissues excised to create pentagonal shape.

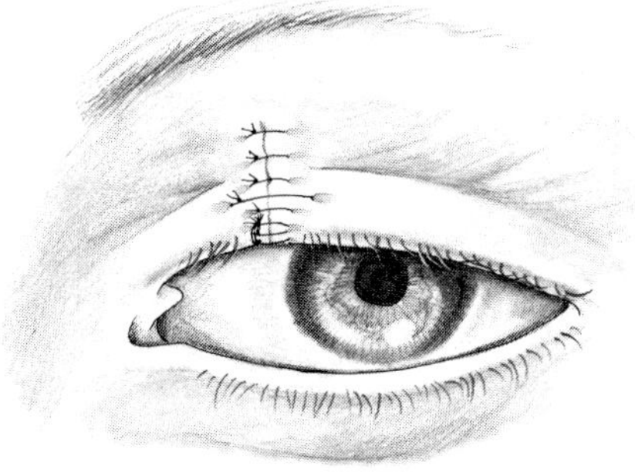

C, Lid margin and cutaneous sutures placed.

Some defects will be too large for direct transmarginal suturing. In these cases, it is possible to relax the tension on the lid with a lateral canthotomy. The canthotomy is begun by crushing the lateral canthus with a hemostat, followed by an incision with scissors (Plate 7-2, *A*). Forceps are used to draw the wound edges together, enabling the surgeon to titrate the amount of dissection required to close the defect.

If the defect cannot be closed with canthotomy alone, additional horizontal relaxation of the lid can be achieved by cantholysis, severing the inferior crus of the lateral canthal tendon. The skin and orbicularis are dissected away from the inferior crus anteriorly, and the conjunctiva is dissected away posteriorly (Plate 7-2, *B*). The isolated inferior crus is severed, with care being taken not to harm the superior crus.

The inferior-crus cantholysis will allow the mobilization of an additional 5 mm of the lateral aspect of the lower lid. The lid defect is closed by the three-suture technique. The lateral canthal incision is closed with 7-0 Vicryl sutures (Plate 7-2, *C*). A pressure patch with antibiotic ointment is placed over the eyelid overnight and removed the next day by the patient. The lid margin sutures are removed 7 to 14 days postoperatively.

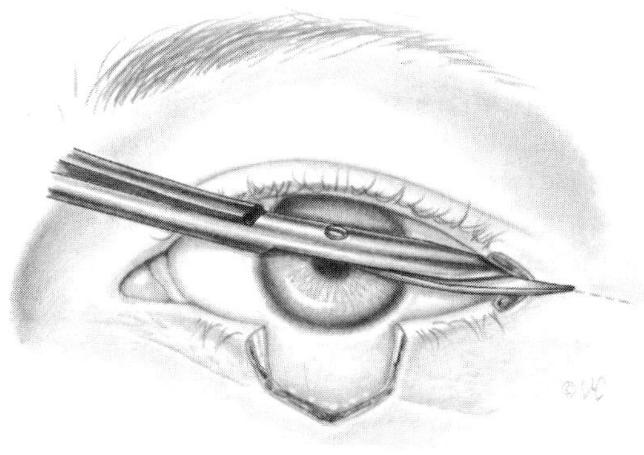

A, Lateral canthotomy performed.

B, Inferior crus cantholysis to lengthen the lower lid.

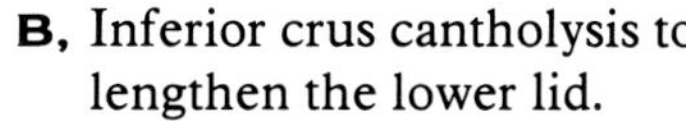

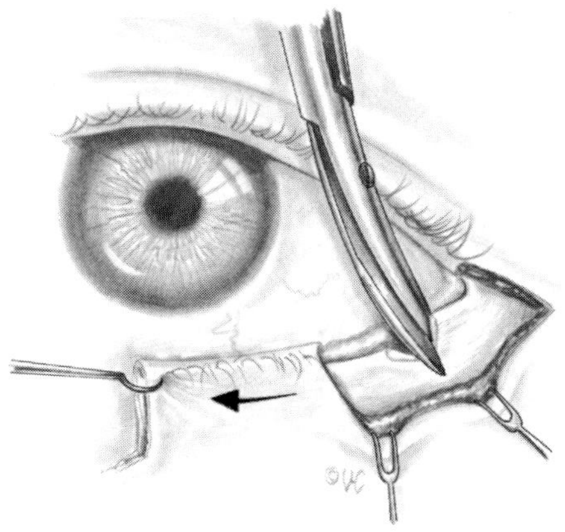

C, Lid defect and lateral canthal incision closed with 6-0 silk and 7-0 Vicryl, respectively.

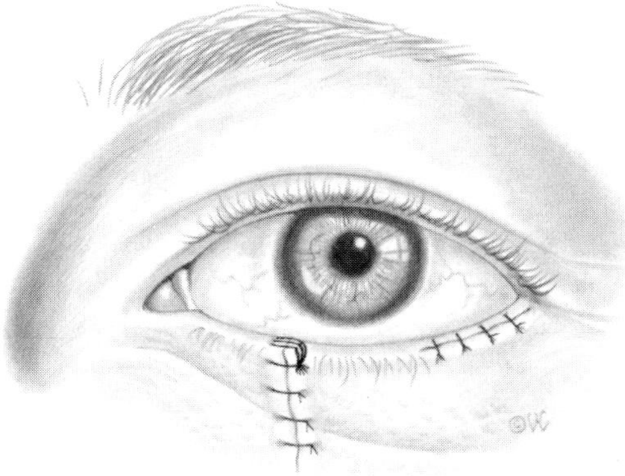

A composite graft is composed of multiple eyelid tissue elements. It can be used to replace full-thickness eyelid defects, such as when a tension-free closure of an eyelid defect cannot be achieved with cantholysis and horizontal advancement of the remaining lid. Its primary advantage over a tarsoconjunctival flap procedure is maintenance of a clear visual axis during surgery in the central eyelid (Plate 7-3, *A* and *B*).

After a lateral cantholysis has been shown to be insufficient to allow direct closure of the residual defect, the contralateral eyelid is examined to determine if there is enough tissue in it to harvest for a full-thickness or composite graft. The graft harvest is begun by making one half of a pentagonal wedge resection. The freed tissue is pulled laterally to confirm that enough eyelid remains for a direct closure, without any residual tension. A lateral canthotomy and cantholysis can be helpful when a large graft is required and its excision would otherwise place residual tension on the wound closure. The donor site is closed with the classic three-suture technique used to close pentagonal wedge resections. Minimal cautery is used on the recipient bed, to promote vascularization of the graft.

The graft is handled very carefully. It is not allowed away from the sterile field. Either the surgeon or the assistant is grasping it at all times. The assistant stabilizes it while the surgeon sutures it into the recipient bed. A 6-0 silk suture is used to stabilize the lid margins by passing it through the meibomian orifices on either side of the graft–recipient bed junction. The tarsal layer is closed with 5-0 Vicryl from the anterior surface (Plate 7-3, *C*). The graft's pretarsal orbicularis is removed (Plate 7-3, *D*), and the skin is closed with interrupted 6-0 mild chromic sutures (Plate 7-3, *E*). Pressure on the graft is avoided. The patient is instructed to use a metal shield at night to protect the graft.

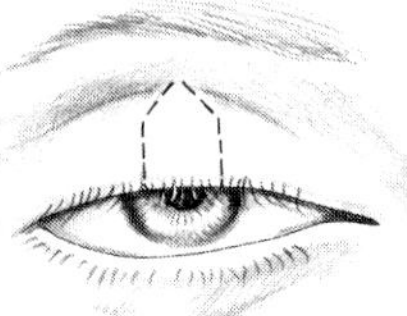 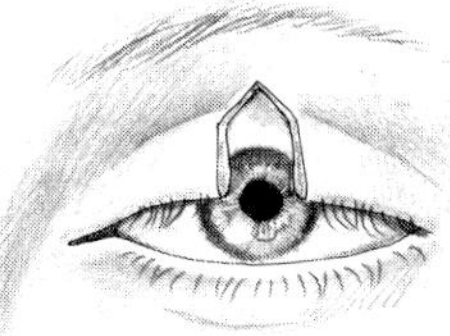

A, Large central defect in left upper lid, with area of composite graft outlined on right upper lid.

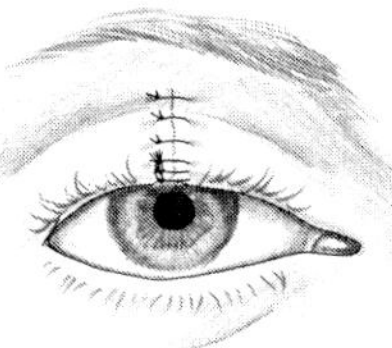 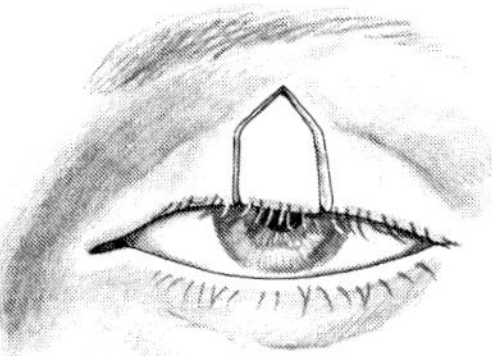

B, Graft placed in defect of left upper lid. Right upper lid closed with three-suture technique.

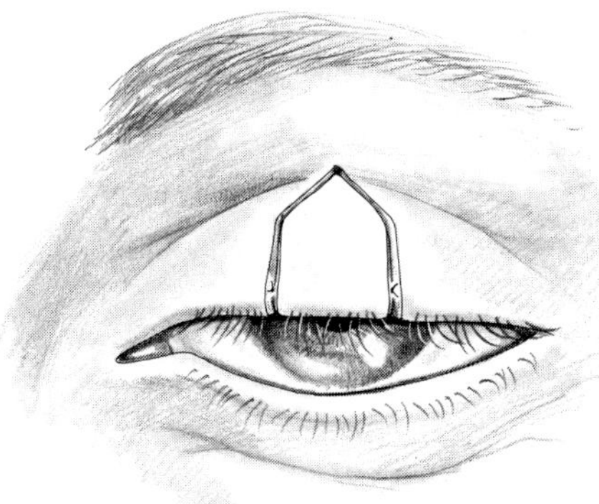

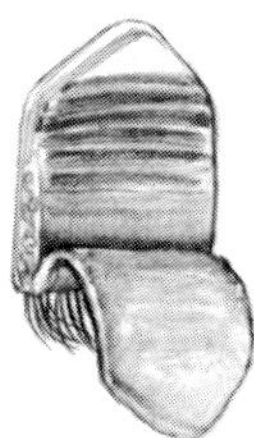

D, Pretarsal orbicularis is removed from the graft.

C, Graft with pretarsal fascial suture in place.

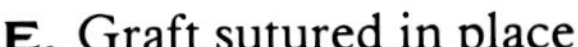

E, Graft sutured in place.

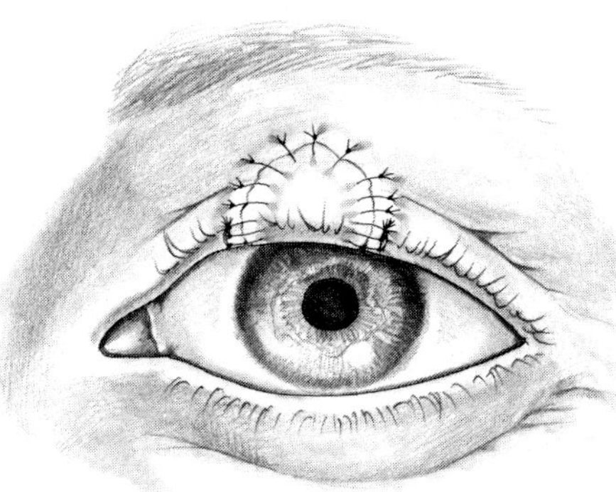

Composite graft with pedicle flap

A composite graft may also be taken from an opposing lid, with a small pedicle being retained. The usefulness of pedicles is probably more theoretic than real, since they are extremely fragile and often slough as a result of pressure necrosis from even a mild insult. For this reason, all dressings are avoided in this technique.

The donor site from which these grafts are taken is located either temporally or nasally to the defect (Plate 7-4, *A*). Following the same technique of lateral cantholysis, the donor graft is incised and rotated gently to fill the defect (Plate 7-4, *B*). The pedicle flap is carefully sutured into place and the donor site closed by the same suture techniques as for the free graft (Plate 7-4, *C*). The pedicle is lysed after a 2- to 3-week interval.

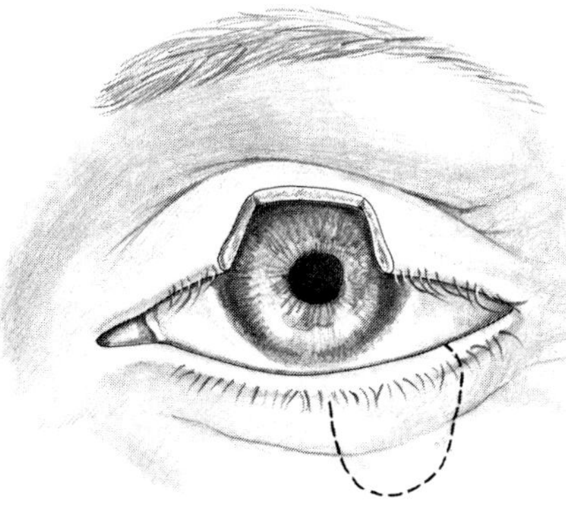

A, Central-lid defect, with lower lid pedicle flap outlined.

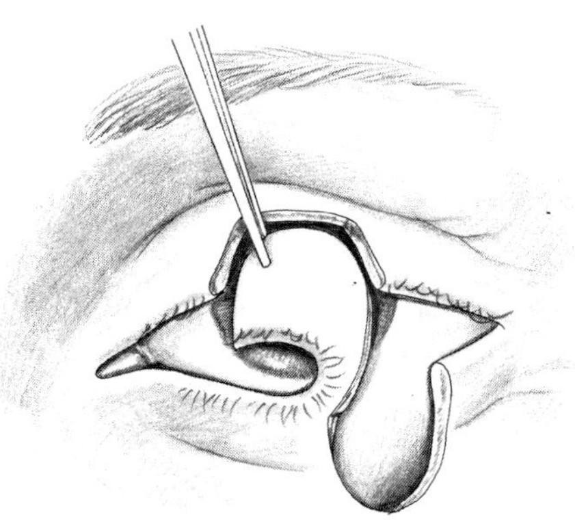

B, Pedicle flap rotated to fill defect.

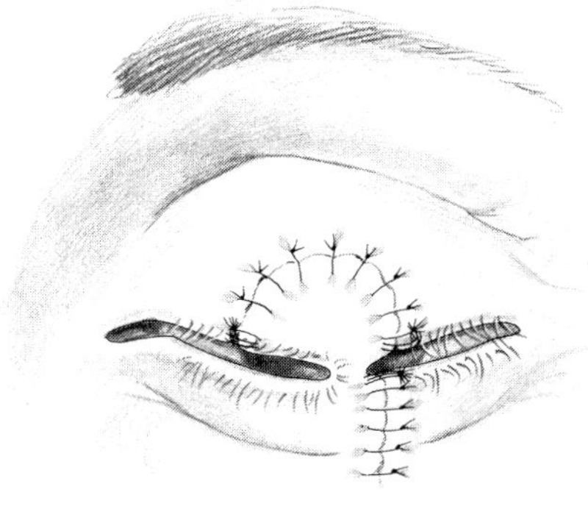

C, Pedicle flap sutured into defect and lower-lid donor site closed.

Semicircular temporal advancement flaps permit mobilization of additional eyelid without the risk involved in using delicate composite grafts and disturbing an otherwise normal eyelid. They offer the advantage of minimizing the horizontal dissection of the temporal area and decreasing the chance of scarring and canthal deformity. They can also be used to fill central defects of up to one half of the eyelid length.

The lateral canthal area is anesthetized with 1% lidocaine with 1:100,000 epinephrine, and the area is allowed to vasoconstrict for several minutes. The lid defect is trimmed to ensure smooth margins and a pentagonal shape. A skin-orbicularis flap is begun at the lateral canthus, extending superiorly and temporally in a crescent fashion (Plate 7-5, *A*). A canthotomy and cantholysis are used to gain access to the canthus, and the skin muscle flap is mobilized (Plate 7-5, *B*).

A conjunctival lining is needed for the posterior raw surface of the flap. It may be obtained by preserving the conjunctiva from the original defect or by using a free tarsal graft, or a free mucous membrane graft. It may be necessary to excise a triangular piece of tissue from the base of the flap to prevent puckering.

The central wound is closed with the three-suture technique. The lateral canthus is closed with a vertical mattress suture, the deep part of which passes full thickness and joins it to the full thickness of the lower-lid tissue. The sutures then unite the new lower lid with the original canthal angle. This suture is tightly secured. The lateral canthal tendon is secured to the back of the skin muscle flap with a 5-0 Vicryl suture (Plate 7-5, *C*). The remainder of the wound is closed with near-far, far-near sutures interspersed with interrupted 6-0 silk sutures (Plate 7-5, *D*). A light dressing is applied.

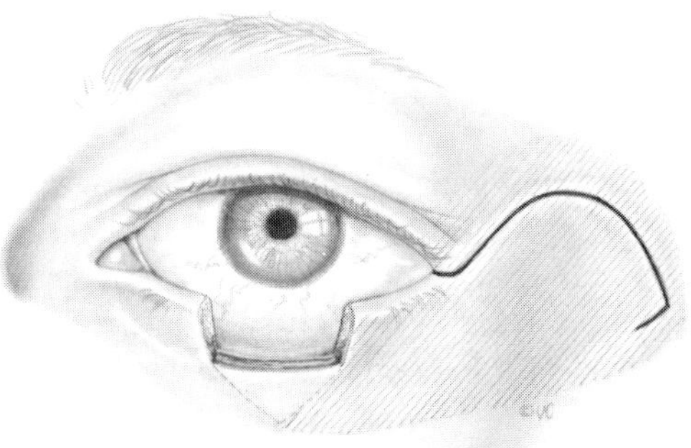

A, Lid defect is trimmed to form pentagon and lateral skin-muscle flap begun.

B, Lateral canthal tendon is lysed and the skin-muscle flap is mobilized.

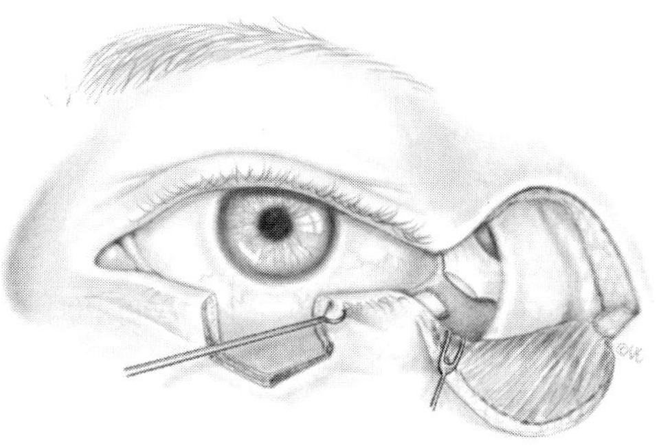

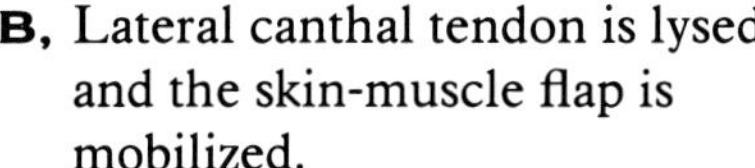

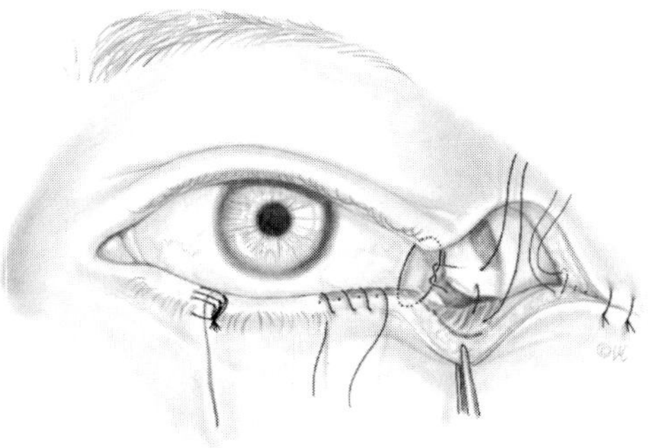

C, Lid margin with 6-0 silk suture. Canthal angle and canthal tendon secured.

D, Lid margin closed with 6-0 silk sutures. Canthal incision closed with 7-0 Vicryl and laterally with 6-0 silk sutures.

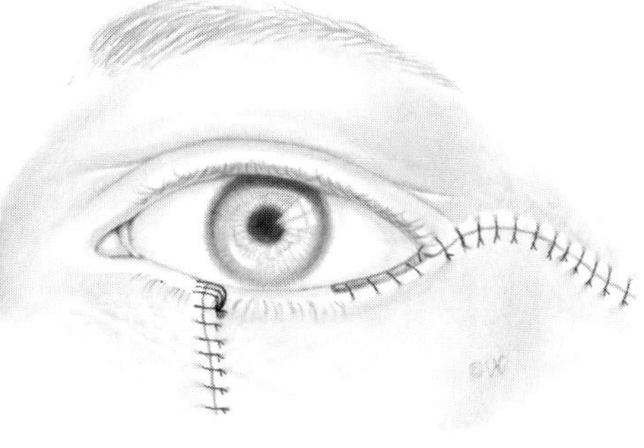

Tarsoconjunctival flaps are the principal method of reconstructing large defects of the lower eyelids. The tarsoconjunctival graft provides the internal lamella of the graft, and the anterior lamella is provided by either a full-thickness skin graft or an advancement skin flap (Plate 7-6, *A* and *B*).

The upper and lower lids are infiltrated with a 50% mixture of 1% lidocaine and 0.75% Marcaine, both with 1:100,000 epinephrine. The lower lid defect is trimmed to provide a smooth, well-defined wound edge. The edges of the defect are brought together gently with forceps to minimize the size of the flap required to fill the defect and to avoid flaccidity of the reconstructed lid. The required flap size is measured with a ruler or calipers. The upper eyelid is everted over a Desmarres retractor, and additional local anesthetic is injected subconjunctivally. The horizontal dimension of the flap is marked on the conjunctiva. A 3-mm-wide strip of tarsus is left along the eyelid margin to maintain support for the upper lid. The incision is made with a razor knife through 80% of tarsus around the length of the proposed flap. Curved iris scissors are used to complete the incision to avoid injury to the orbicularis. The dissection is carried sufficiently far superiorly to allow the tarsoconjunctival graft to rest in the lower lid defect without residual tension.

The horizontal borders of the recipient tarsus are grooved to receive the newly created flap, and the inferior border of the flap is sutured to the base of the recipient bed with 6-0 Vicryl sutures (Plate 7-6, *C*). A double-armed, 6-0 silk suture is used to attach the horizontal edge of the recipient bed to the flap in a vertical mattress fashion. Both needles are passed through the conjunctiva and tarsal plate of the lower eyelid posterior to the grooves created to receive the flap. They are brought out through the posterior surface of the groove and passed full thickness through the tarsoconjunctival flap. Both needles are then passed through the anterior surface of the groove and out through the skin surface (Plate 7-6, *D*). The suture is brought through the skin well away from the incision edge to avoid pressure on the incision by the bolster. The flap is pulled snugly into position with the 6-0 silk suture, which is then tied over a rubber-band bolster. At this point, the flap is sutured firmly into place on all three sides.

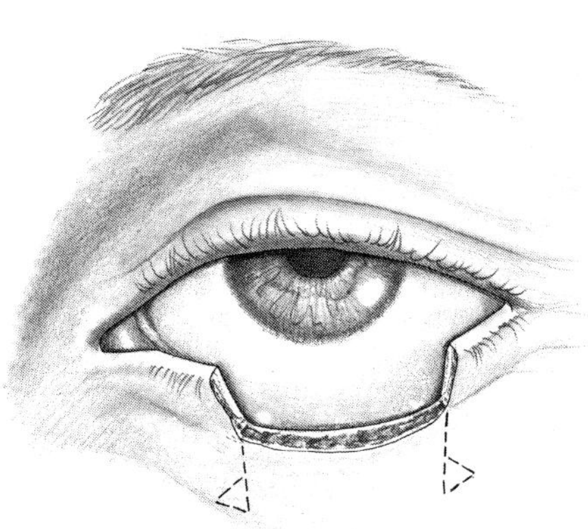

A, Large central defect, with outline of external advancement flap.

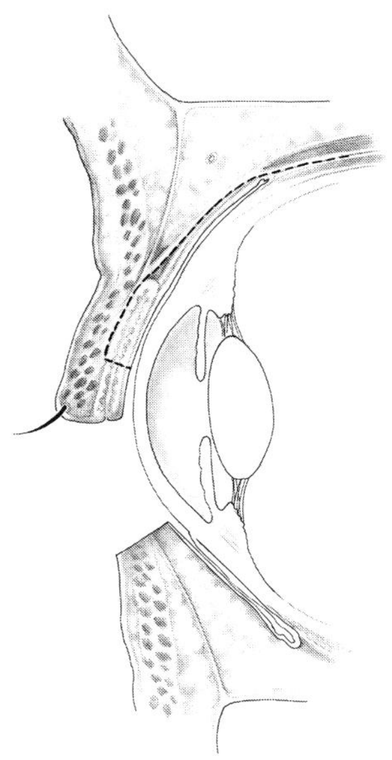

B, Sagittal section demonstrating outline of advancement flap.

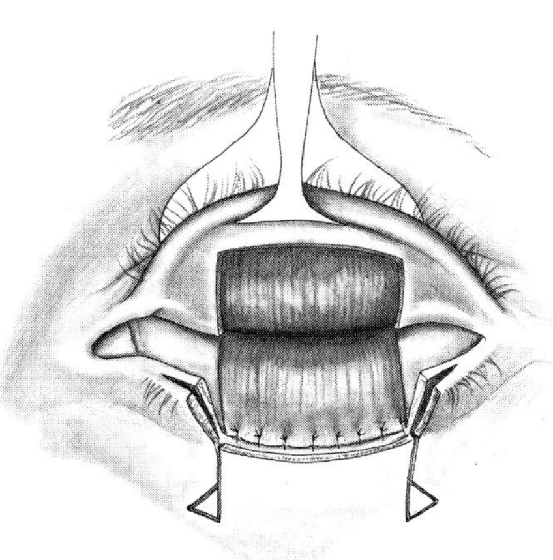

C, Everted lid with advancement flap dissected and sutured into defect. Lower-lid grooves created to receive edges of flap.

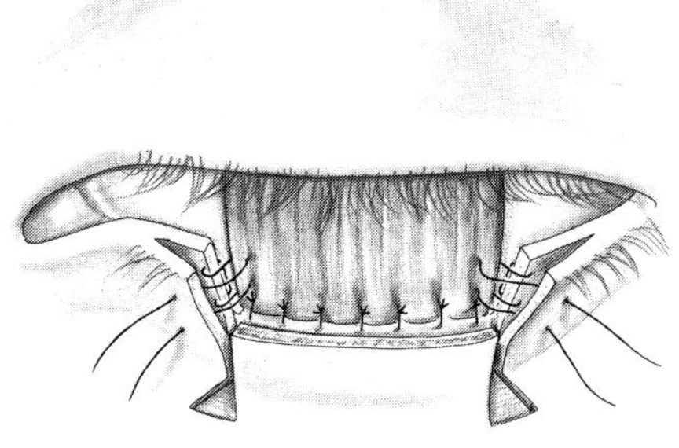

D, Insertion of mattress suture to pull tarsus into grooves.

A sliding skin flap is ideal for covering the anterior surface of the tarsoconjunctival flap. The flap is created by making vertical incisions through the skin only and dissecting it sufficiently far inferiorly to avoid vertical shortening of the lower eyelid when the flap is advanced into position. The orbicularis is not included in this flap, to minimize the risk of postoperative lid retraction. Two triangular excisions are made at the base of the flap to create a smooth junction (Plate 7-6, *D*). The graft should be pulled superiorly with minimal tension. The incision is closed with interrupted 6-0 mild chromic suture. The superior border of the skin flap is attached to the tarsoconjunctival flap at the superior border of the tarsus with interrupted 7-0 Vicryl sutures (Plate 7-6, *E*). If there is not sufficient lid skin available for this type of advancing flap without creating a vertical lid retraction, a free skin graft is required to cover the graft. The free skin graft may be obtained from a contralateral lid, the retroauricular area, or the supraclavicular area. It is harvested in the previously described fashion and secured in place with interrupted 6-0 mild chromic sutures along the inferior and lateral margins. The superior border of the skin graft is attached to the superior border of the tarsoconjunctival graft's tarsal plate with interrupted 7-0 Vicryl suture (Plate 7-6, *F* and *G*).

The conjunctival bridge is opened in 3 to 6 weeks. The timing is determined by the graft's postoperative appearance. The graft is severed 1 mm above the desired lid margin with scissors after a blunt instrument is placed posterior to the graft to protect the eye (Plate 7-6, *H*). The resulting lid margin is sculpted smooth with thermal cautery. The remaining conjunctival stump is trimmed to avoid irritation and vertical shortening of the upper eyelid.

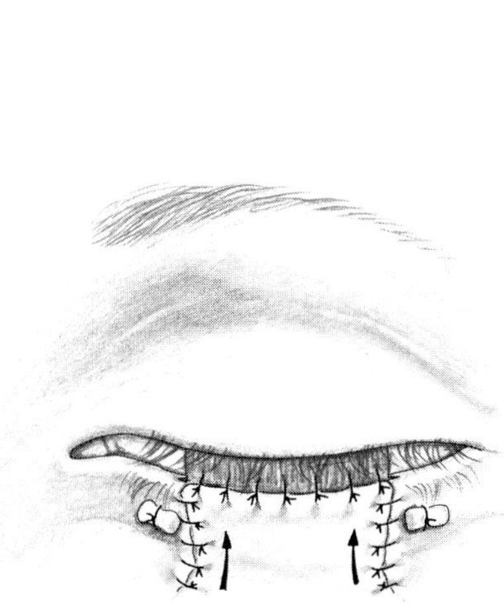

E, Advancement of external flap to cover graft.

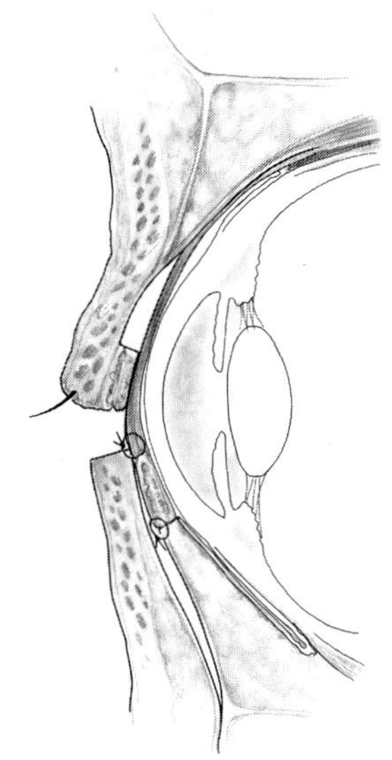

F, Sagittal view of tarsoconjunctival flap covered with advancement flap.

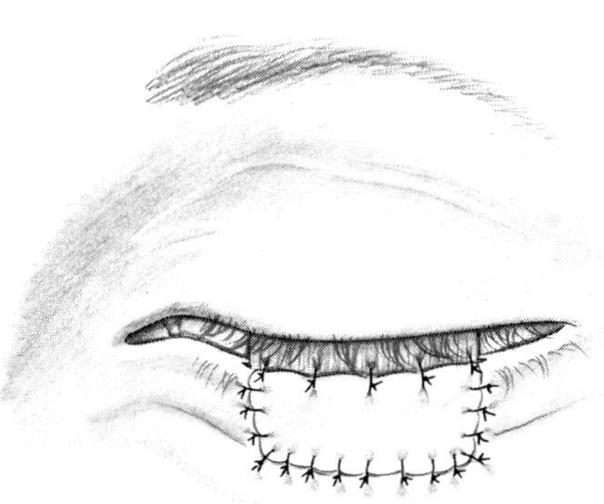

G, Free skin graft used in place of advancement flap.

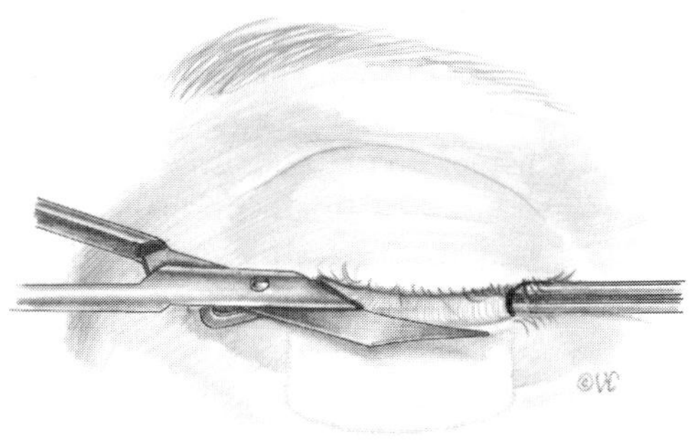

H, Opening of tarsorrhaphy.

A full-thickness bridge flap can be utilized for repairing large central defects of the upper lid. As we have seen, the techniques of lateral canthotomy and cantholysis, composite grafting, and semicircular advancement flaps can all be used for the repair of upper-lid defects. However, when the defect is so large that even the combination of more than one of these procedures is insufficient, we prefer the bridge flap over those procedures that require rotation flaps hinged on a narrow pedicle. This involves the full substance of the lower lid in preference to procedures using horizontal advancement flaps of the lateral canthal area, which are better suited for lower-lid repair.

Following the injection of suitable anesthetic in the lid, the full-thickness upper-lid defect is trimmed to ensure smooth edges while sacrificing as little as possible of the healthy lid tissue. A marking pencil is used to delineate a base-down flap 4 mm below the lash line. The width of the flap should be the size of the defect to be filled (Plate 7-7, *A*).

With a bone plate or other suitable flat instrument behind the lower lid, the anterior surface of the flap is incised over the marked area. Care must be taken to remain 4 mm from the lash line to avoid damaging the marginal arterial arcade. The incision should include skin alone. The lid is everted and a separate incision made through conjunctiva and tarsus to be in apposition with the anterior incision. Curved iris scissors are used to connect the two incisions. This is done to avoid angling the flap edge, which may cause damage to the arterial arcade.

The surgeon uses the scissors to extend the dimensions of the flap horizontally until the desired width is achieved. From the ends of the incision, full-thickness vertical incisions are created down to the lower fornix. Both the flap and the bridge must be handled gently to avoid compromising the circulation. It is useful to handle the bridge by means of thin, soft rubber tubing passed under it rather than with instruments.

The bridge flap, freed from any attachments on three sides, is now gently passed under the marginal bridge. The conjuctiva and Müller's fibers of the upper lid are sutured to the conjunctiva of the advancement flap with 7-0 Vicryl sutures (Plate 7-7, *B*). The levator aponeurosis and septal layer of the upper lid are joined to an ear cartilage graft with 6-0 Vicryl sutures. The ear cartilage graft is harvested as discussed above and trimmed to size (Plate 7-7, *C*). The skin-muscle layer is closed with interrupted 6-0 silk sutures. Therefore the flap passes under the marginal bridge and extends upward to join the base of the defect in the upper lid, where it is anastomosed (Plate 7-7, *D*). The posterior surface of the flap protects the eye (Plate 7-7, *E*). The inferior edge of the bridge flap is left to reepithelialize on its own, with no sutures used, to avoid undue pressure. A Telfa strip, with an appropriate area for the bridge removed, is applied and covered with a light gauze dressing. Superficial sutures are removed after 4 to 5 days.

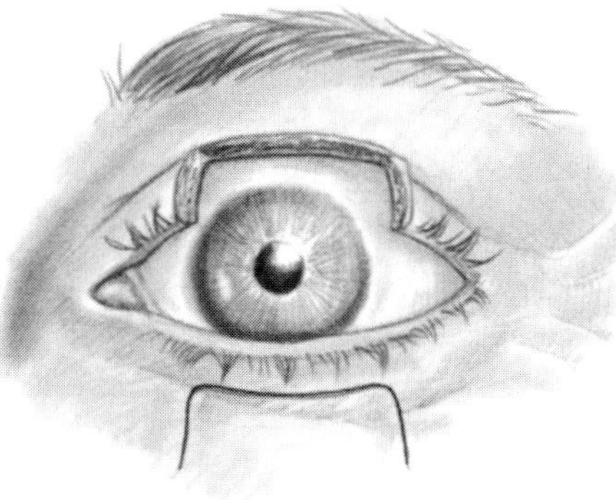

A, Large central upper-lid defect, with outline of full-thickness lower flap.

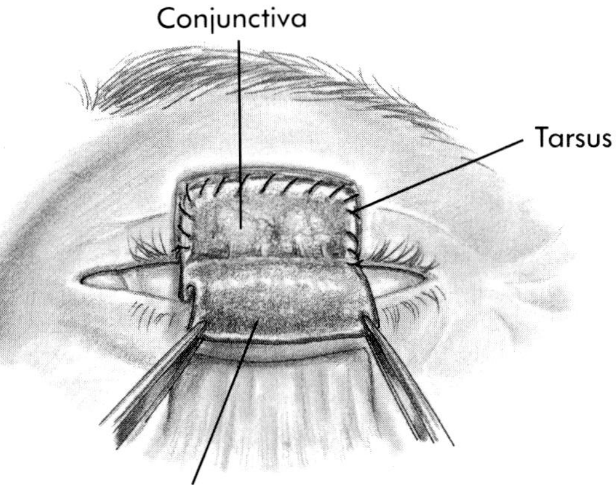

B, Conjunctival layer closed with 7-0 Vicryl suture.

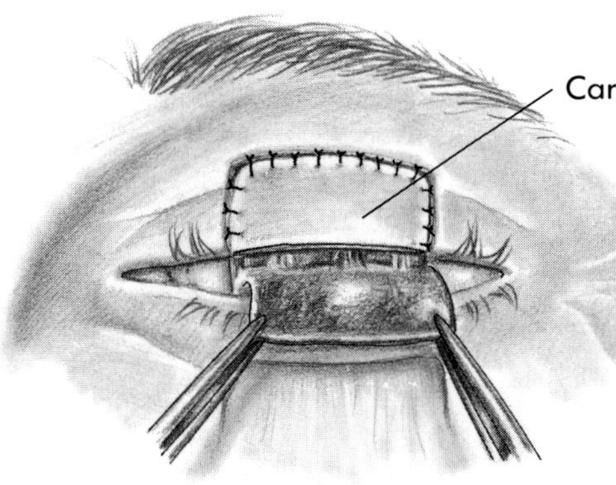

C, Ear graft trimmed and sutured into place with 6-0 Vicryl suture.

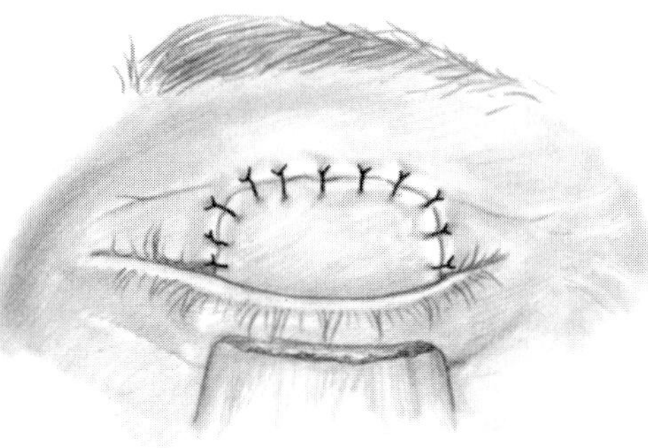

D, Skin-muscle layer closed with 6-0 silk suture.

After a 6- to 8-week interval, during which time the flap stretches to almost double its length, the tarsorrhaphy is opened. A protective instrument is placed under the flap, and it is incised with a knife blade. The lower edge of the newly created lid will epithelialize on its own. The lower edge of the marginal bridge is denuded and sutured to the upper edge of the skin flap. The lower lid should be in the original position with no vertical deficit, and the upper lid should be of good contour (Plate 7-7, *F*).

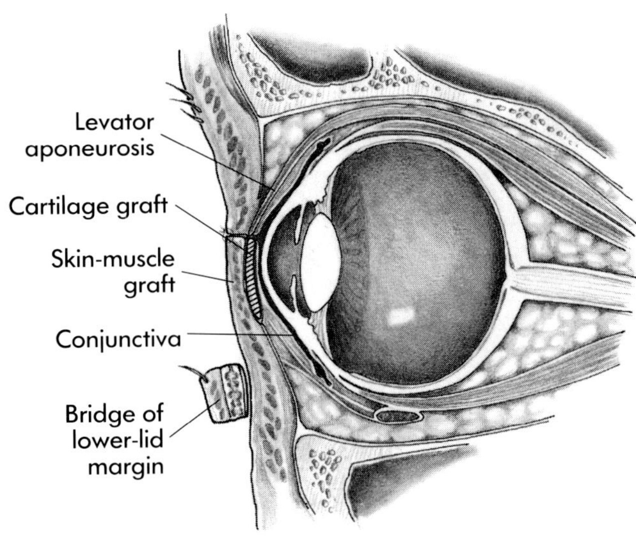

E, Sagittal section demonstrating advancement flap under marginal bridge with sutures in place.

F, Bridge flap severed and reattached to lower lid. Margin of upper lid sutured closed.

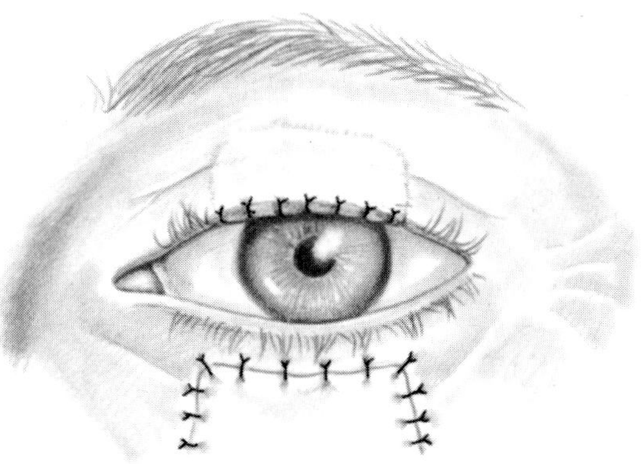

The Mustardé technique is a procedure particularly suited for replacement of an entire upper lid. It requires considerable experience in the technique and handling of large dissections. The ophthalmologist who does not have the skill and training to perform such procedures should probably call on the expertise of a surgeon trained in facial plastic work. A poor result with this procedure means considerable facial distortion and potential loss of both upper and lower lids. This procedure is presented here so that the surgeon will have some familiarity with the handling of as extensive a problem as complete upper-lid loss. General anesthesia is usually preferred with this procedure because of the extent of the dissection. However, infiltration with local anesthetic containing epinephrine is done to minimize intraoperative bleeding.

A curvilinear incision is begun at the lateral canthus, arching superiorly and temporally and then down in front of the ear. The lower crus of the lateral canthal tendon is then released. A skin muscle dissection is completed so that the cheek flap is ready for rotation. Just temporal to the punctum, a full-thickness lid incision is made into the lower fornix, and the entire lower lid is released at the level of the inferior orbital rim, with a small pedicle left attached at the lateral canthus. The area below the excised lid is carved into a triangular shape (Plate 7-8, *A*).

A piece of nasal septal cartilage is then obtained. The cartilage obtained should have nasal mucosa on one side of it. The cartilage is trimmed to fill the inner lamellar defect now present in the lower lid. The mucosal side of the graft faces the globe. The remaining conjunctiva in the lower lid is sutured with 6-0 chromic catgut sutures to the mucosa. The cartilage is secured to the remaining tarsus laterally and to orbicularis inferiorly with 5-0 Vicryl sutures (Plate 7-8, *B*).

The cheek flap is then rotated medially and the lower eyelid brought into position to fill the upper lid defect (Plate 7-8, *C*). The pedicle must be treated gently, because it contains the marginal artery needed for survival of the flap. The conjunctival layer (nasal mucosa) of the new lower lid is sutured with 6-0 Vicryl sutures to the edge of the cheek flap. The cheek flap is closed with 6-0 nylon sutures.

In the new upper lid the conjunctiva of the flap is sutured to the conjunctiva of the defect with fine absorbable sutures. The levator, septum, and orbicularis are approximated to the flap structures. The skin is closed with 6-0 mild chromic interrupted sutures. A light dressing is applied to avoid necrosis to the pedicle. Superficial sutures are removed after 4 to 5 days. The pedicle is severed after 3 weeks and the lid margins are revised (Plate 7-8, *D*).

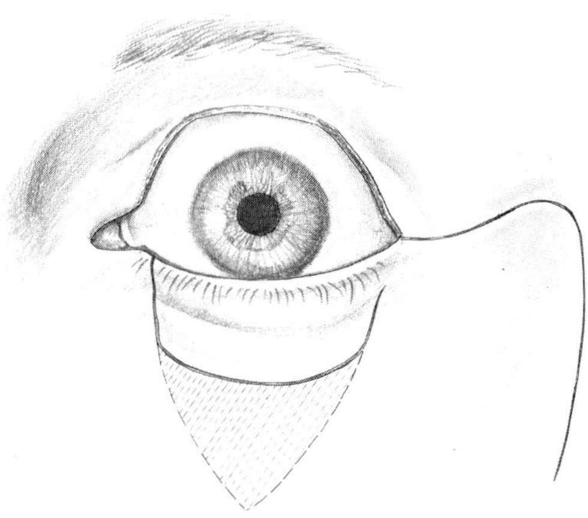

A, Deficiency of entire upper lid, with dissection of temporal curvilinear rotation flap and release of entire lower lid.

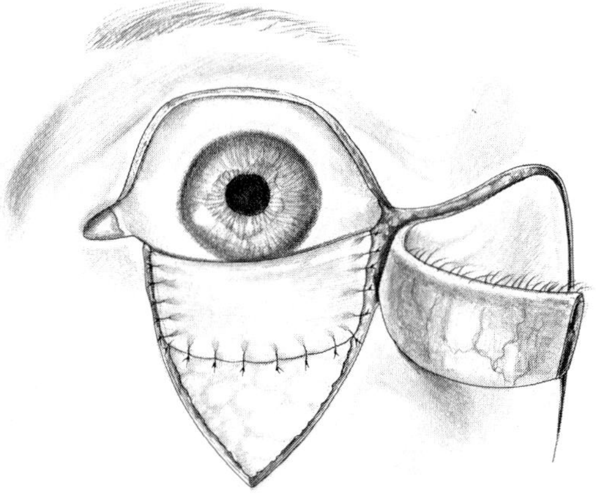

B, Nasal septal cartilage sutured in place of tarsoconjunctival flap.

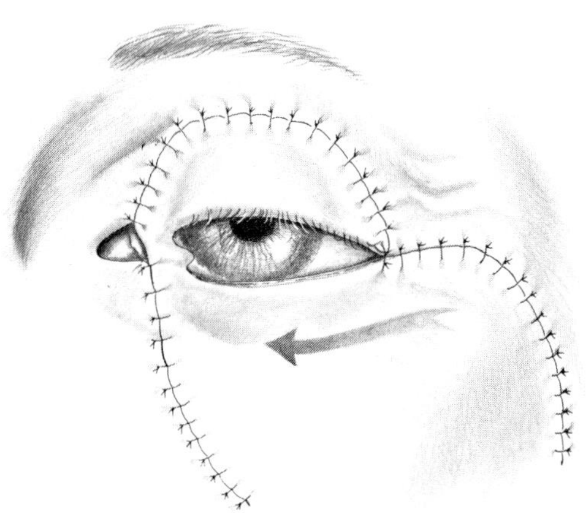

C, Curvilinear flap rotated nasally while lower lid transposed superiorly.

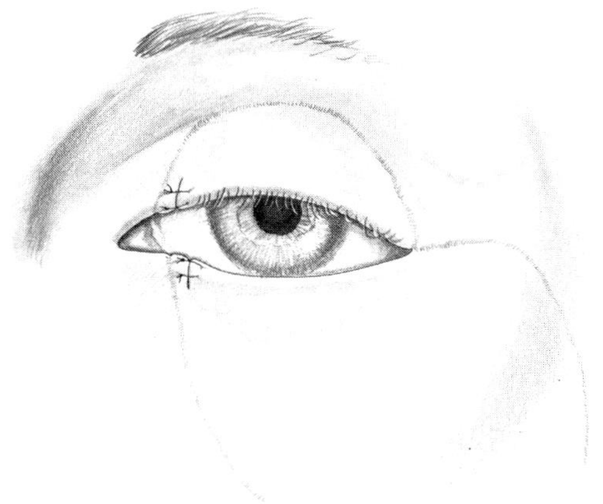

D, Interpalpebral band lysed and lid margin revised.

Temporal advancement flaps are suitable as a means of lower lid replacement and, if the defect is small enough, can be used without replacing the inner lamella of the lid. However, the usual reason for using this type of flap is that the defect is of such a magnitude that simpler and more direct means of lid closure are insufficient. Therefore it is necessary to use a free tarsal, nasal cartilage, or buccal mucous membrane graft to line the flap.

Although we prefer a procedure in which upper-lid donor material is advanced to fill the defect, the procedure can be used to fill defects greater than one-half the length of the lid. The area is infiltrated with a 50:50 mixture of 2% lidocaine and 0.75 Marcaine, both with 1:100,000 epinephrine.

A large central defect in the lower lid should be trimmed to a pentagonal shape (Plate 7-9, *A*). Beginning at the lateral canthus, an incision is made superiorly and temporally. The inferior crus of the lateral canthal tendon is lysed at its insertion to the lateral orbital tubercle. A skin-muscle flap is dissected temporally. If a defect greater than one half the length of the lid is to be filled, the incision is curved downward in front of the ear and a cheek rotation flap created.

The temporal flap is advanced. The marginal wound is closed with the three-suture technique. The raw edge of the flap is lined as necessary. The temporal wound is closed with interrupted 6-0 mild chromic sutures (Plate 7-9, *B*). The lateral canthus is closed with a vertical mattress suture.

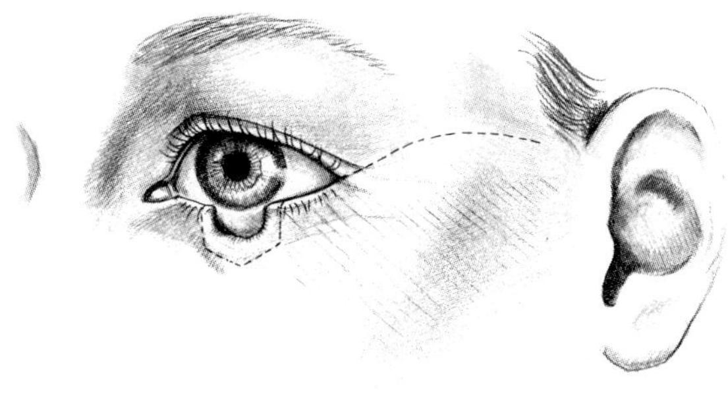

A, Large central defect with outline of pentagonal incision and temporal flap.

B, Flap advanced and sutured into defect and wound closed with interrupted sutures.

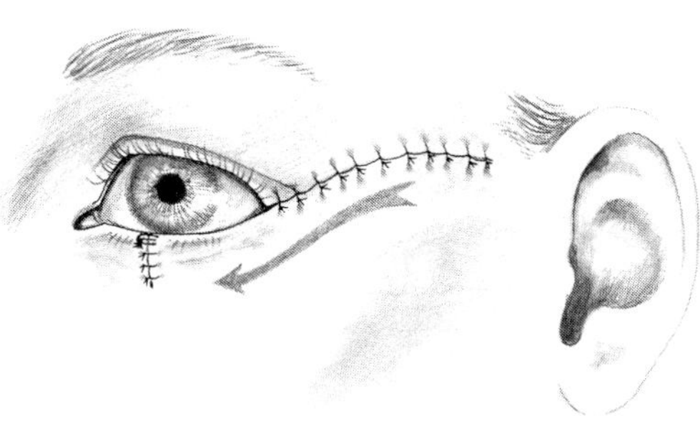

The external layer of the lower lid may be contracted as a result of superficial traumatic, chemical, or thermal injury. The temporal transposition flap is particularly useful for the replacement of the skin and orbicularis layers of the lid, when the internal layers are viable. A free skin graft may also be used in this area. However, if the defect extends beyond the lateral canthus and subcutaneous tissue is excised, a depression may result.

A horizontal incision is made along the superior aspect of the fibrotic area, parallel to the lid margin. The skin and underlying tissue retracting the lid are dissected free and excised. The defect is trimmed to a workable contour (Plate 7-10, *A*). A strip of gauze is held at the temporal end of the dissection and rotated upward to ascertain the limits of the flap, which are outlined with a marking pencil.

The vertical transposition flap is incised and, beginning at its apex, dissected to include skin and enough subcutaneous tissue to include a vascular bed. If the length of this flap is greater than 2½ times its width, its transposition should be delayed, as previously described. The base of the flap is sufficiently undermined to permit its easy transposition.

The donor bed is closed by extensive undermining of the adjacent wound edges and the use of 4-0 nylon near-far, far-near sutures interspersed with interrupted 6-0 nylon sutures. If the wound is wide enough, subcutaneous suturing with absorbable sutures may be necessary. Hemostasis may be achieved with thermal cautery in the donor bed.

The surgeon sutures the flap into place with interrupted 6-0 mild chromic sutures, first orienting it into position with the extremities secured (Plate 7-10, *B*). Hemostasis should be achieved in the recipient area with moderate pressure rather than cautery. The area superior to the base of the flap is not sutured, because pressure might compromise the circulation in the flap. This area will granulate closed. It may be revised as needed at a later date.

A light Telfa dressing is applied. Superficial sutures are removed after 4 to 7 days and near-far, far-near sutures 3 to 7 days later. Adhesive strips are then applied for about 1 week to the donor site. Three weeks following the initial surgery the base of the flap may be released and that area modified. The flap tends to be thickened for several weeks until the edema subsides. Further modification should be delayed until 6 months later.

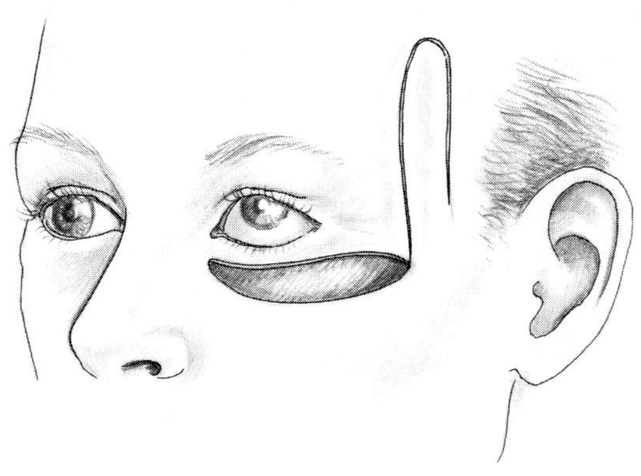

A, Temporal transposition flaps. Horizontal incision made through skin and subcutaneous tissue and subsequent dissection to release lower lid. Temporal flap dissected. Note presence of subcutaneous tissue.

B, Temporal flap transposed and sutured into defect. Donor site closed with near-far, far-near sutures.

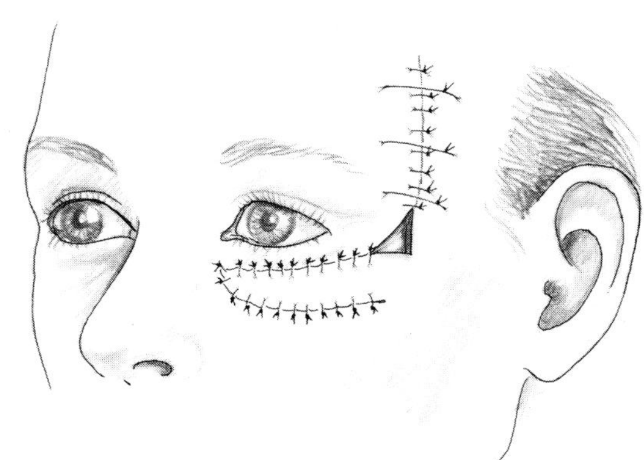

It is our opinion that the procedure of choice in the repair of large defects of the upper lid is the use of a pedicle bridge flap from the ipsilateral lower lid. However, in cases in which there has also been substantial loss of lower-lid tissue, making that lid unsuitable as a donor site, the use of transposed pedicle flaps is indicated. Since these flaps replace the full thickness of the lid, it is necessary to line them with mucous membrane. Although nasal cartilage is suitable for this purpose, it is also possible to line the pedicle flaps with buccal mucous membrane before its transposition.

This is an especially useful technique when the lid defect, although of full thickness, does not involve the margin of the lid with its tarsal plate. Here a mucous membrane lining is required, but the rigidity of nasal cartilage is not necessary.

A marking pen is used to outline the area of the donor flap after a gauze strip has been used as a measuring device to estimate the size and location of the flap (Plate 7-11, *A*). The transposition flap is incised and dissected to a depth that will ensure the presence of a good vascular bed. The flap is dissected from its apex toward the base.

The mucous membrane graft is then obtained. With the lower lip everted on an appropriate clamp or two towel hooks, the inside of the lip is injected with 1% lidocaine with 1:100,000 epinephrine. A Castroviejo mucotome is then used to obtain a graft that is 0.5 mm thick (Plate 7-11, *B*). The clamp is removed from the lip and wet gauze is placed over the wound.

The mucous membrane is immediately transferred to a piece of Gelfilm. The graft is stapled to it with a small stapling device, with its smooth side toward the Gelfilm. The Gelfilm with the attached mucous membrane is trimmed to two-thirds the length of the transposition flap and to an equal width.

The graft stapled to the Gelfilm is then sutured with 4-0 chromic sutures to the subcutaneous part of the transposition flap, with the raw surface of the mucous membrane toward the underside of the flap. The flap is replaced in its bed and sutured with 6-0 silk sutures to allow for longitudinal vascularization and adherence of the graft (Plate 7-11, *C*). A light dressing is applied. The 6-0 silk sutures are removed after 4 days.

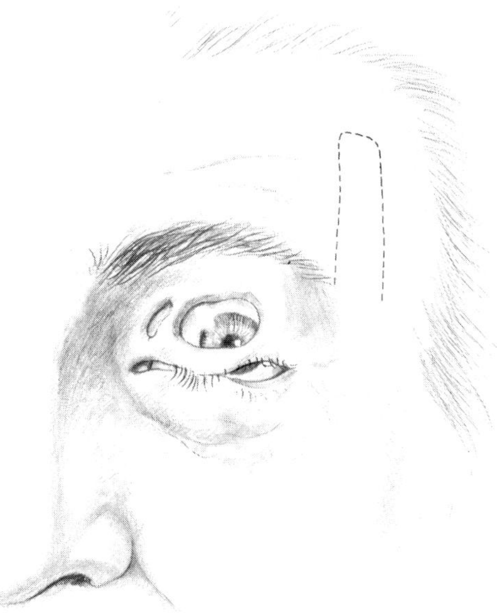

A, Large fistulizing defect of upper lid, with outline of delayed pedicle flap.

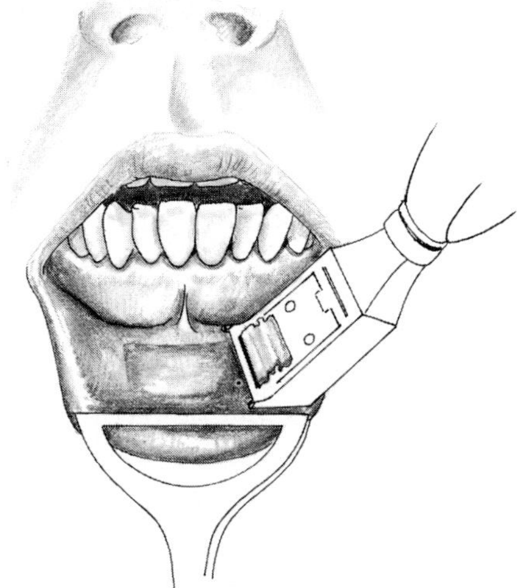

B, Castroviejo mucotome used to obtain donor mucous membrane.

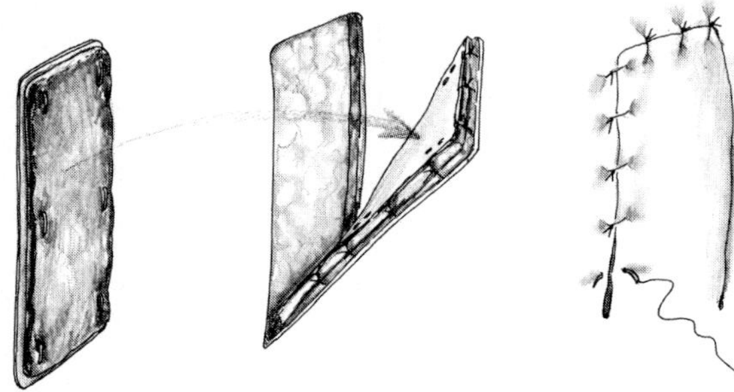

C, Mucous membrane stapled to Gelfilm and sutured to underside of flap. Flap resutured into original position.

After 4 weeks, the second stage of the procedure is performed. The recipient area is trimmed to the approximate size of the transposition flap it is to receive. A knife is used to incise the flap, and blunt dissection is used to reach the level of the mucous membrane. The flap is raised and the Gelfilm carefully removed (Plate 7-11, *D*).

At that time the base of the flap is sufficiently dissected to allow for easy transposition. The donor site is closed, as previously described, with undermining and the use of near-far, far-near sutures.

The flap is closed in layers. The mucous membrane is sutured with 7-0 Vicryl suture to the remaining conjunctiva. The orbicularis layer, which is sutured to the subcutaneous layer of the flap, is closed with 5-0 chromic suture. The skin is closed with interrupted 6-0 mild chromic sutures. Once again, the triangle at the base of the flap is allowed to granulate (Plate 7-11, *E*). A marginal suture is placed from the lower lid margin and anchored to the brow.

A light gauze dressing is applied. The superficial sutures are removed after 4 to 7 days. The near-far, far-near sutures and the marginal suture are removed after 7 to 10 days. Three weeks following the transposition, the base of the flap can be lysed and the area modified.

The flap tends to remain edematous for several weeks. Occasionally, a procedure is needed to thin the flap. Scar revision and dermabrasion, if needed, are delayed until several months after surgery.

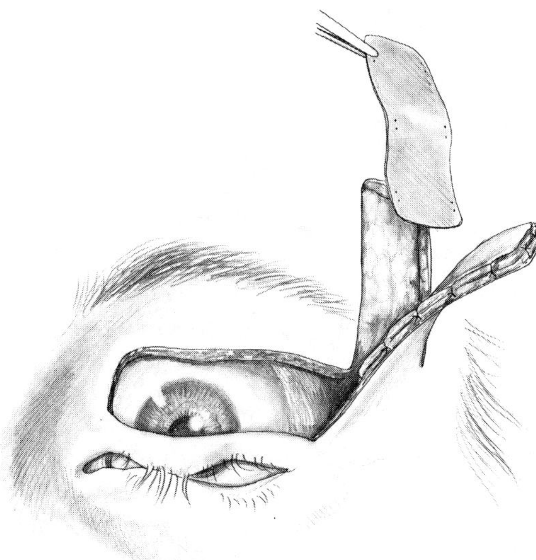

D, Upper-lid fistulas excised. Temporal flap raised and Gelfilm removed.

E, Flap transposed and sutured into position. Marginal lid suture placed. Donor site closed.

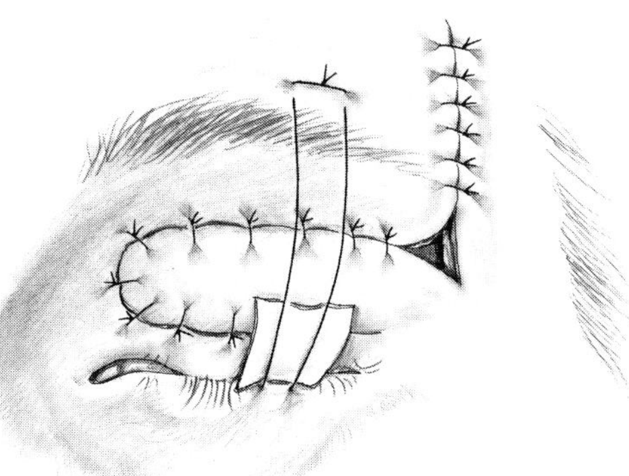

The need for reconstruction of the lateral canthus is generally secondary to lesions that involve the substance of both the upper and lower lids at the lateral canthal angle. Basal cell carcinoma, a common cause of defects in this area, responds poorly to other forms of treatment, and complete surgical excision is the only sure form of therapy. We recommend that lesions in this area be excised widely and deeply. Frozen sections should be obtained to confirm complete extirpation of the tumor.

The initial incisions through the lid are perpendicular to the lid margin (Plate 7-11, *A*). These are carried vertically to the fornices and then turned temporally to circumscribe the lesion. The canthus is rotated outward so that the depth of the excision can be ascertained (Plate 7-12, *B*). Lesions in this area will often require excision down to periosteum. If there is periosteal involvement, this tissue also must be excised.

The specimen should then be completely removed and properly oriented and labeled on a piece of Telfa or other suitable background. The margins of the lesion are examined by the pathologist as separate specimens, including the base of the tissue. Having been reasonably assured following frozen section examination that the margins are clear, the surgeon can proceed to reconstruct the area.

The upper lid is everted and stabilized with a traction suture or an appropriate lid clamp or both. An incision is made with a razor knife 3 mm from the lid margin through the conjunctiva and tarsus wide enough to fill the lateral defect.

The medial end of this incision is extended high into the fornix. With iris scissors the tarsoconjunctival flap is dissected in a plane between Müller's fibers and the levator aponeurosis. When the dissection has been carried sufficiently high into the fornix so that the flap can be easily transposed without causing an arching of the upper lid, the lateral transposition is made. The inferior edge of the flap is sutured to the remaining conjunctiva of the lower lid with 7-0 Vicryl suture. The temporal edge of the lower lid is grooved, and a 6-0 silk vertical mattress suture is passed from inside the lid, through the medial aspect of the flap, to be withdrawn on the skin surface (Plate 7-12, *C*). The overlying skin of the lateral canthus is undermined, and sliding advancement flaps are prepared.

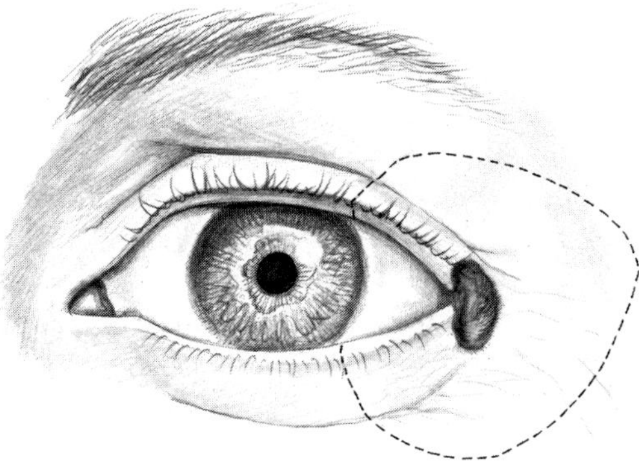

A, Malignant lesion of lateral canthus, with outline of area to be excised.

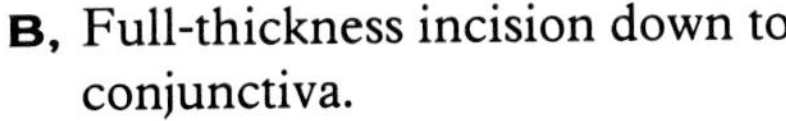

B, Full-thickness incision down to conjunctiva.

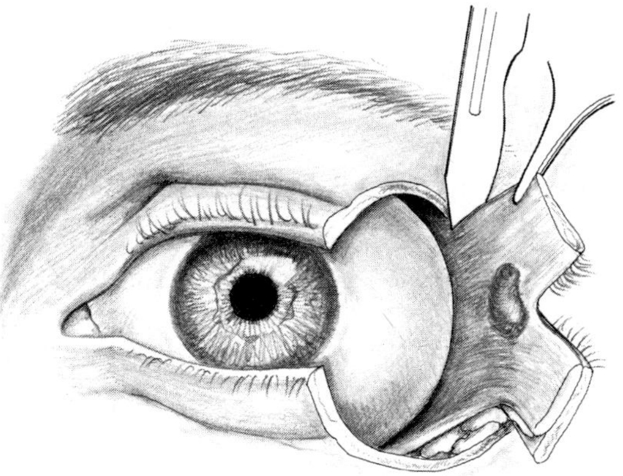

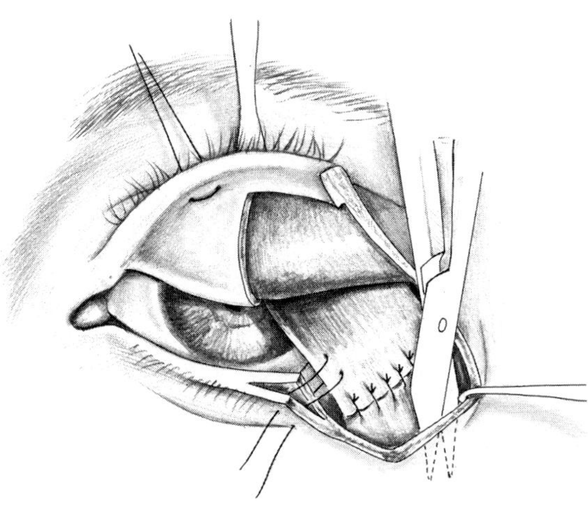

C, Tarsoconjunctival flap transposed from upper lid and sutured into defect. Note mattress suture through intramarginal groove. Adjacent skin being undermined.

A trapdoor flap is now made from periosteum at the lateral canthus. If periosteum has been taken, holes can be drilled into bone for this purpose. A 6-0 silk mattress suture is placed from this flap through a groove slot that is created in the medial aspect of the upper lid. The lower-lid mattress suture is then tied over a rubber-band bolster (Plate 7-12, *D*).

The initial suture through the new canthal tendon is also tied over a rubber-band bolster, and more absorbable sutures are placed to secure this to the flap. The sliding skin flaps are then advanced at the lateral canthus (Plate 7-12, *E*). The surgeon closes the skin layer with interrupted 6-0 mild chromic sutures, trimming the skin flap where necessary (Plate 7-12, *F*). A light dressing is applied and changed daily for several days. The mattress sutures are removed after 1 to 2 weeks.

Following a 3- to 6-week period, the tarsorrhaphy is severed. The wound edges are sculpted with thermal cautery and sutured at the new mucocutaneous junction with 7-0 Vicryl sutures.

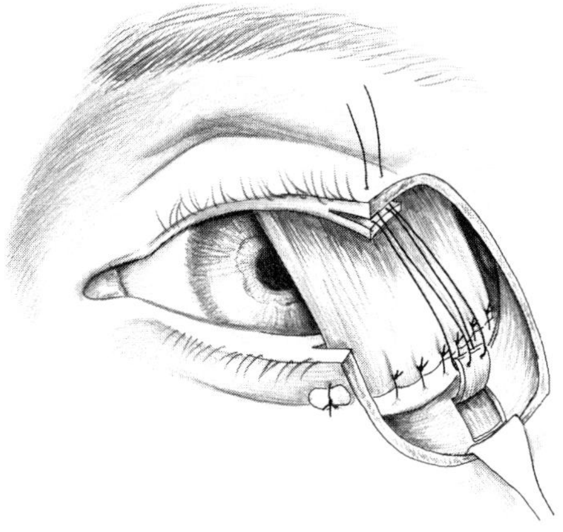

D, Periosteal hinged flap being created and sutured to upper lid to recreate lateral canthal tendon.

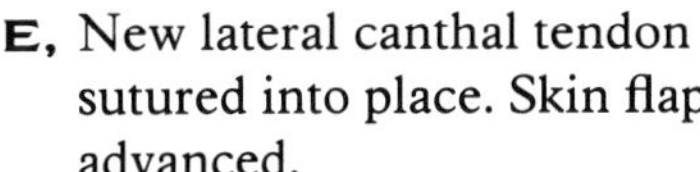

E, New lateral canthal tendon sutured into place. Skin flap advanced.

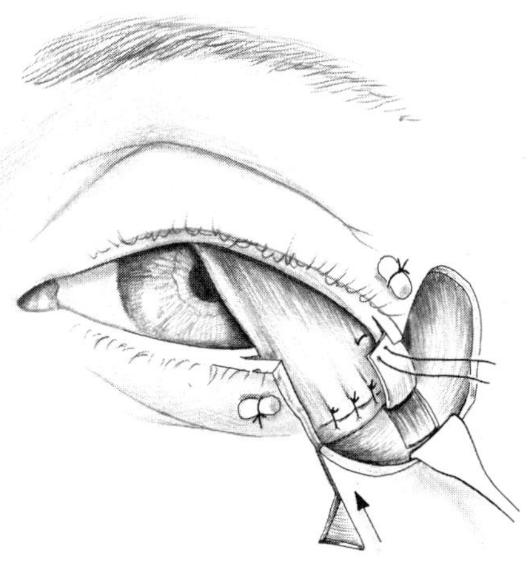

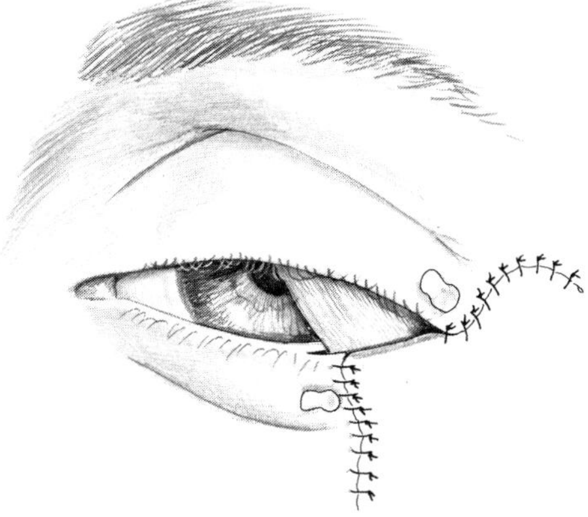

F, Skin closure with interrupted 6-0 mild chromic suture.

The excision of lesions in the medial canthus requires reconstructive techniques that generally are more involved than those at the lateral canthus. The anatomy of this area is more complex, with the presence of the medial canthal tendon and the lacrimal system. If the complete excision of the lesion requires removal of these elements of the lacrimal system, then not only must the anatomic configuration of the lids and medial canthal angle be reconstituted, but the lacrimal drainage system must also be recreated.

Generally, at the time of surgery the area that is to be excised is outlined with a surgical marking pen (Plate 7-13, *A*). The initial perpendicular incisions through the lid margins are made through an area in which the architecture of the meibomian orifices is intact. Distortion and obliteration of these orifices are evidence of invasion of this area.

The incisions are extended to the fornices and then turned horizontally to widely circumscribe the mass. The angular vessels are usually encountered at the canthal angle, and hemostasis is achieved with bipolar cautery. At this point the surgeon determines by visual examination or frozen section if the lacrimal structures need to be excised. If so, the dissection is extended down to periosteum (Plate 7-13, *B*). The main specimen is sent to the pathologist for en bloc permanent sections. Peripheral strips of tissue are sent for frozen section. This segregation of specimens is used to minimize the chance for confusion between the surgeon and the pathologist.

For the surgeon who performs this operation infrequently, closure of most canthal defects is probably best achieved by awaiting gradual granulation of the area. This technique enables the surgeon to concentrate on the complete eradication of the lesion without the worry of a complicated reconstructive procedure.

After the excision has been completed, the lids are closed and held together with interrupted 6-0 silk sutures tied over a cotton bolster (Plate 7-13, *C*). This area is packed with a petrolatum dressing and then covered with a loose gauze dressing. The loose dressing is changed daily, with great care not to disrupt the new granulating tissue. The petrolatum dressing is removed and changed every 3 to 4 days. After complete granulation has occurred, the medial canthal angle may need to be surgically modified.

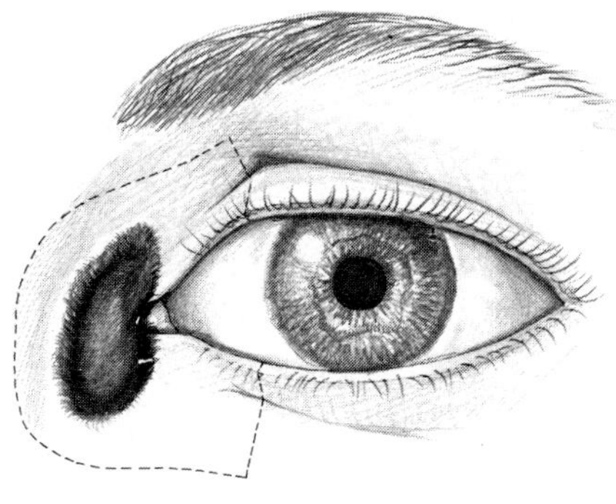

A, Large medial canthal lesion involving lacrimal excretory system. Area to be excised outlined.

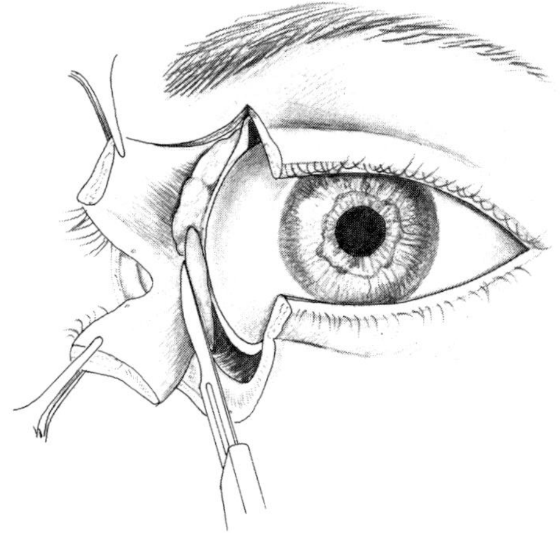

B, Dissection extended down to expose full extent of lesion.

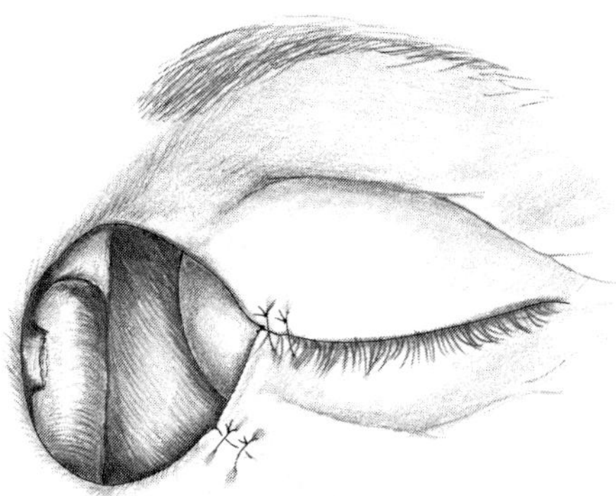

C, Lids closed and sutured together.

For the more experienced surgeon, the area can be reconstructed with a tarsoconjunctival graft taken from the upper lid. The upper lid is everted and reflected temporally. A razor knife is used to incise the conjunctiva and tarsus 3 mm from the lid margin (Plate 7-14, *A*). The incision is extended temporally to create a flap about the size of the defect to be filled. The dissection is made sufficiently high into the cul-de-sac, between the tarsus and the retractors of the upper lid (levator aponeurosis and Müller's muscle), to allow its medial transposition.

The tarsoconjunctival flap is then brought down into position into the lower fornix and sutured to what remains of the conjunctiva with 6-0 Vicryl sutures. The stump of the medial canthal tendon, if it remains, is sutured to the tarsoconjunctival graft with 5-0 nylon sutures (Plate 7-14, *B*). If the medial canthal tendon stump is not present, then the graft is sutured with 5-0 (35-gauge) stainless steel wire to the anterior lacrimal crest after this has been drilled with several holes.

Next, the surgeon prepares the lower lid to receive the tarsoconjunctival graft by creating a groove in it, into which interdigitates the inferolateral aspect of the graft (Plate 7-14, *C*). A 6-0 silk vertical mattress suture is used, woven from the inside out to hold this area in position, as previously discussed.

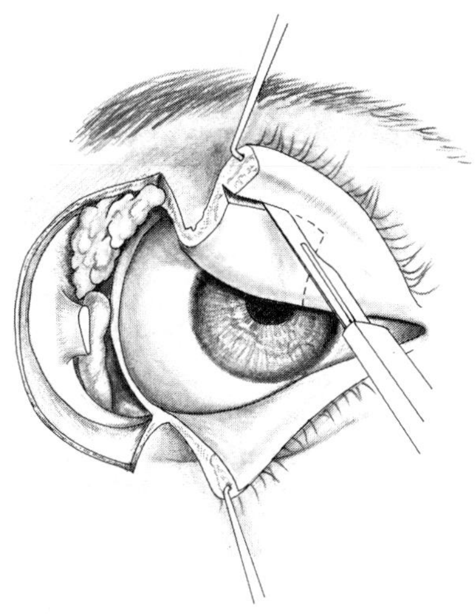

A, Preparation of tarsoconjunctival flap. Note 3 mm area of lid margin preserved.

B, Flap transposed and sutured into position. Stump of medial canthal tendon sutured to tarsal flap.

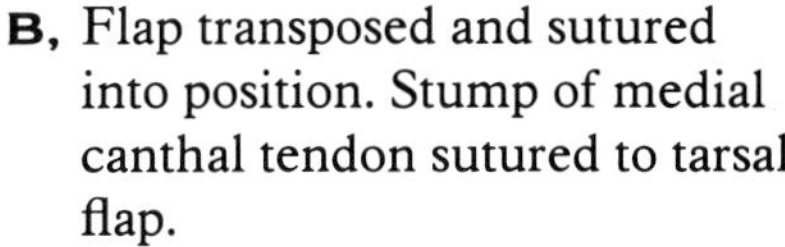

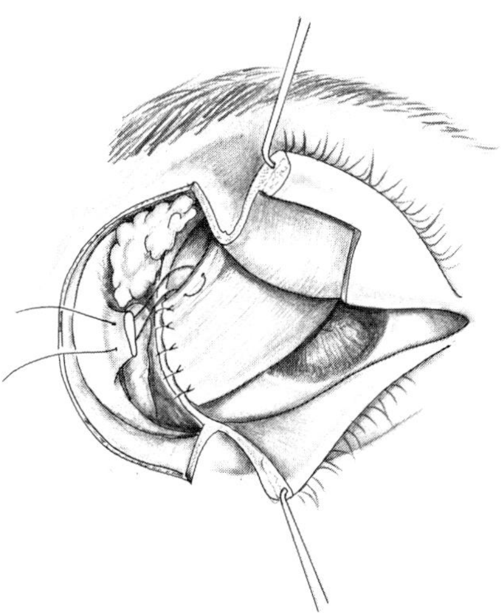

C, Medial canthal tendon recreated. Graft being sutured into lower lid groove.

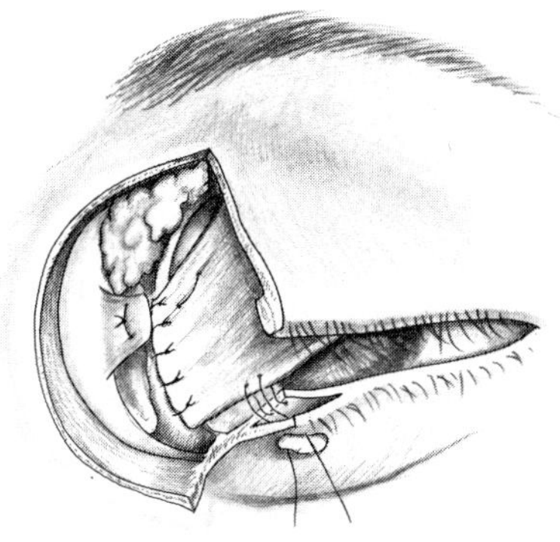

The closure of the overlying wound is best achieved by the use of a free full-thickness skin graft. There is no readily available skin for the creation of advancement flaps in the medial canthal area. Therefore full-thickness skin from the contralateral upper lid, or a retroauricular graft as a second choice, is an excellent match for the medial canthal area.

The skin graft is cut to the shape of the defect (Plate 7-14, *D*) and sutured into place with interrupted 6-0 mild chromic sutures. The suture ends are left about 1½ inches long. The graft is then perforated with multiple "pie crust" incisions to prevent fluid accumulation beneath it.

The suture ends, which have been left long, are tied over a cotton or Telfa bolster. (Plate 7-14, *E*). A 6-0 silk Frost suture is generally placed and tied over pledgets to keep the lid in position for approximately 4 to 5 days. The bolster is removed after 3 days and the silk suture after 5 to 6 days. With the packing secured over the graft, a light dressing is applied.

The surgeon must be careful to begin the initial incision 2 to 3 mm from the lid margin, or an entropion may result. If the tarsoconjunctival graft is stretched to reach the recipient area and not dissected high enough into the cul-de-sac, arching of the lid will result. "Rounding" of the medial canthal angle is a possibility and may need to be modified later with a medial canthoplasty. Fluid accumulation beneath the skin graft may result in sloughing of the graft. Care must be taken to incise the graft and to apply gentle pressure with a nonadhesive dressing, as described above.

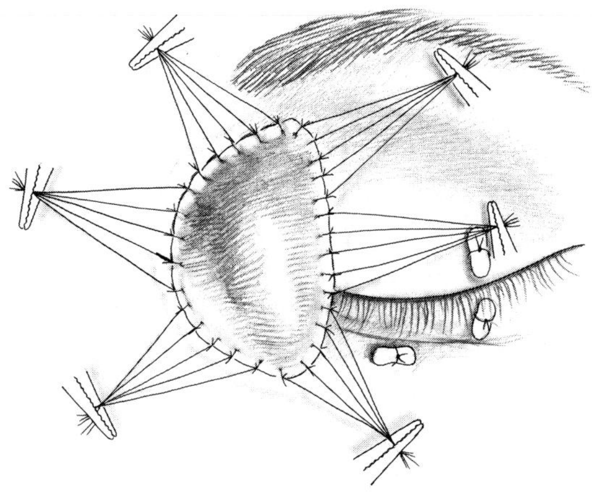

D, Free skin graft placed over defect.

E, Bolster tied over graft with suture ends.

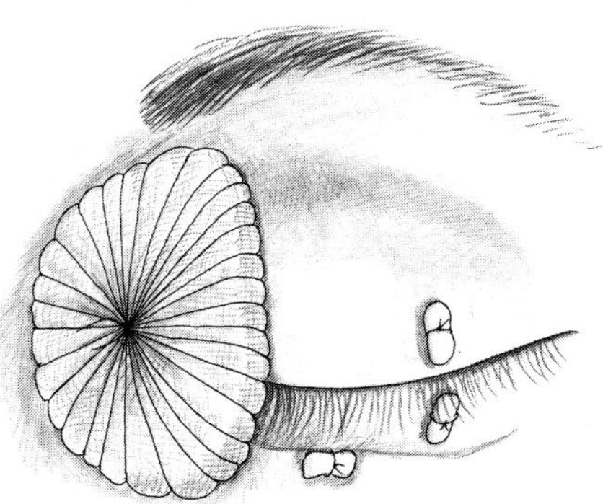

ENTROPION REPAIR

Entropion is the inward rotation of the eyelid margin. It causes significant ocular irritation and can cause visual loss resulting from corneal opacification. Entropion is divided into two broad categories, cicatricial and noncicatricial. Cicatricial entropion can be caused by any condition that results in conjunctival scarring. It is usually a progressive problem, and several surgeries over many years may be necessary to control the progressive shortening of the posterior eyelid lamellae. Eyelid laxity is not a significant contributing factor in cicatricial entropion. Noncicatricial, or involutional, entropion is caused by horizontal and vertical eyelid laxity. The horizontal lid dimension may be increased and may need to be decreased by a tarsal strip procedure, a triangular tarsal resection, or a pentagonal wedge resection. The capsulopalpebral fascia is usually detached from the inferior border of the lower lid tarsus. Eventually, the preseptal orbicularis overrides the pretarsal orbicularis, causing the lid margin to rotate inward. Reattaching it will rotate the lid margin outward as well as enhance the lid rigidity. Most cases of noncicatricial entropion will benefit from a combination of horizontal shortening of the eyelid (see Chapter 9) and reattachment of the capsulopalpebral fascia.

A chalazion clamp is placed at about two-thirds the distance from the medial to the lateral canthus (Plate 8-1, *A*). The clamp should be sufficiently large to expose the full dimension of the tarsus. Using a razor knife, the surgeon outlines a triangle, with its base at the lower tarsal margin and its apex about 2 mm from the lid margin. The triangle should be incised through the conjunctiva and down to the tarsus (Plate 8-1, *B*). The base of the triangle is 7 to 10 mm in length. The triangle is excised with the razor knife, with dissection extended down to the pretarsal orbicularis.

Following the incision of this tarsoconjunctival base-down triangle, three to four 5-0 Vicryl sutures should be placed across the defect so that when tied the knots will be buried within the wound (Plate 8-1, *C*).

Before the sutures are tied, the chalazion clamp should be loosened and the sutures tied from the base upward (Plate 8-1, *D*). The chalazion clamp is then removed. A small elevation of the lid margin is usually present, but disappears within a few weeks (Plate 8-1, *E*). The sutures are left to be absorbed, but could be removed after 7 days if necessary.

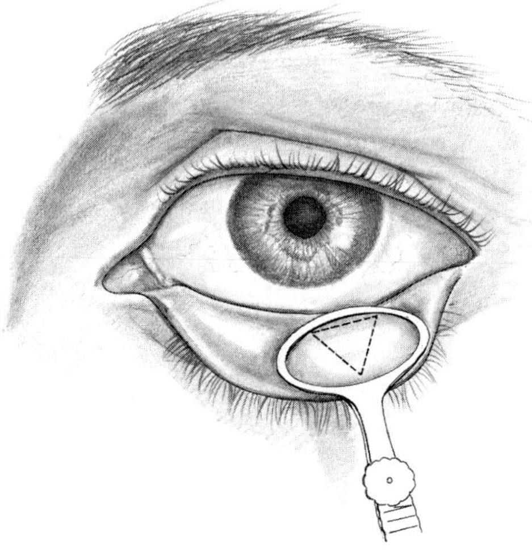
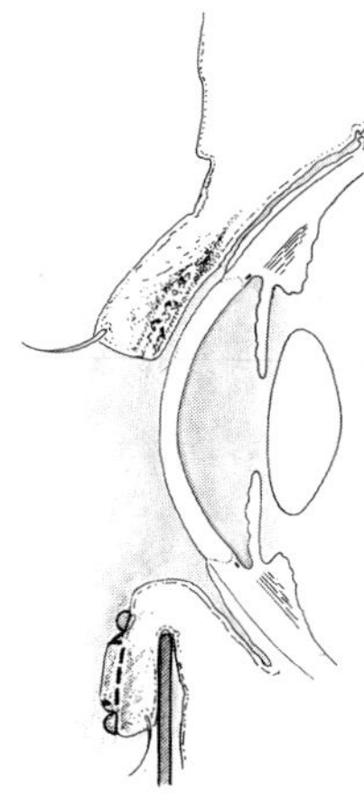

A, Chalazion clamp placed on lower lid, with area to be resected outlined.

B, Sagittal section to show depth of incision.

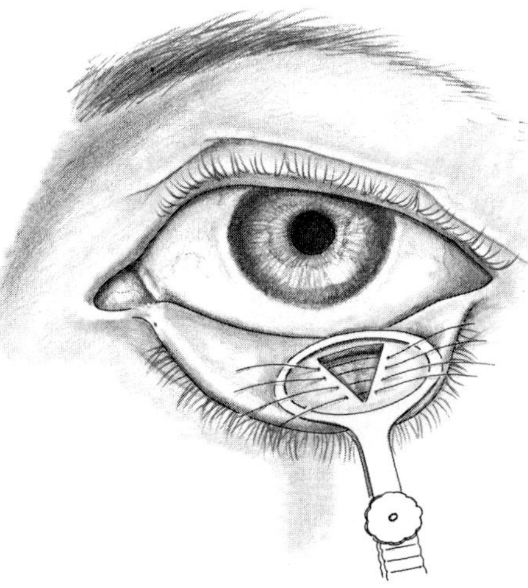
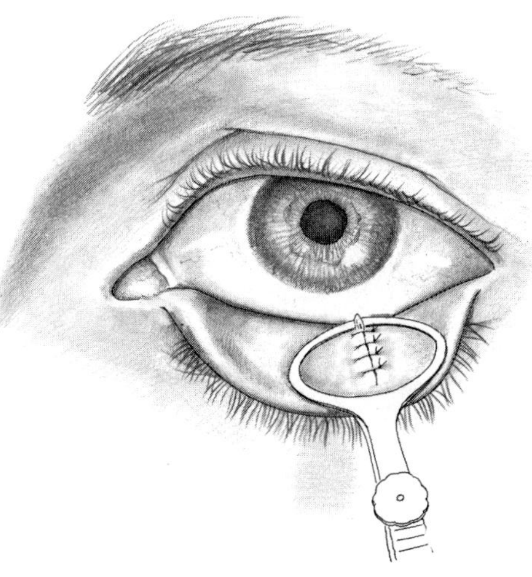

C, Sutures placed across surgical defect in tarsus.

D, Clamp loosened and sutures tied.

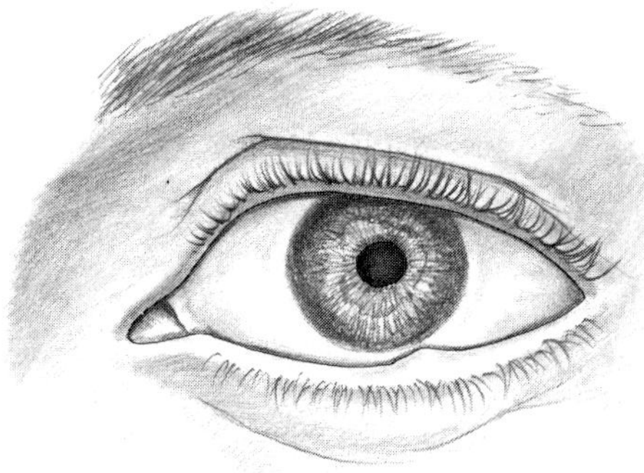

E, Lid position at end of procedure. Note small elevation of lid margin.

A strip of orbicularis is dissected free through a subciliary blepharoplasty incision. The temporal end of the strip is transposed and attached to the periosteum of the inferior orbital rim, thus physically extra-rotating the lid margin and at the same time causing a scarring between the pretarsal orbicularis, the preseptal orbicularis, and the underlying tissue.

A marking pen is used to create a line 2 to 3 mm below the lash line, extending from just below the punctum to the temporal smile crease (Plate 8-2, *A*). The area is infiltrated with 2% lidocaine with 1:100,000 epinephrine, for lid akinesia and hydraulic dissection. A razor knife is then used to incise along the demarcated line. A lid plate may be used for protection during this step (Plate 8-2, *B*).

The skin overlying the lower lid is dissected free from the orbicularis muscle with curved iris scissors and Castroviejo forceps. The dissection is carried down to the inferior orbital rim (Plate 8-2, *C*).

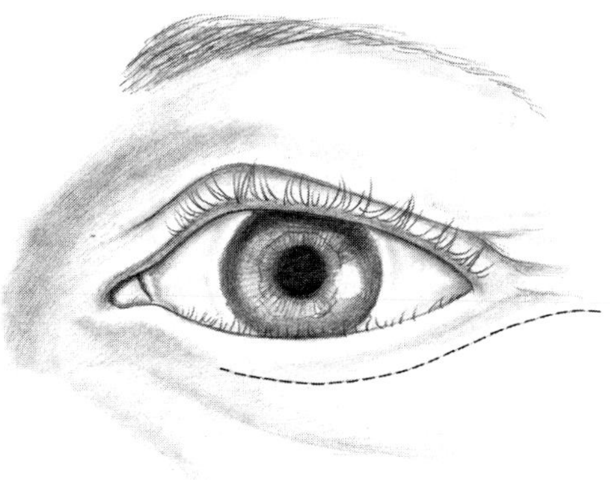

A, Outline of subciliary incision to be made.

B, Lid plate in place and skin incision being made.

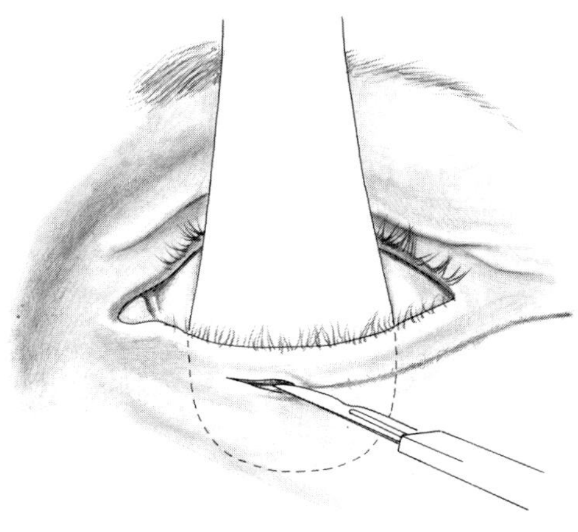

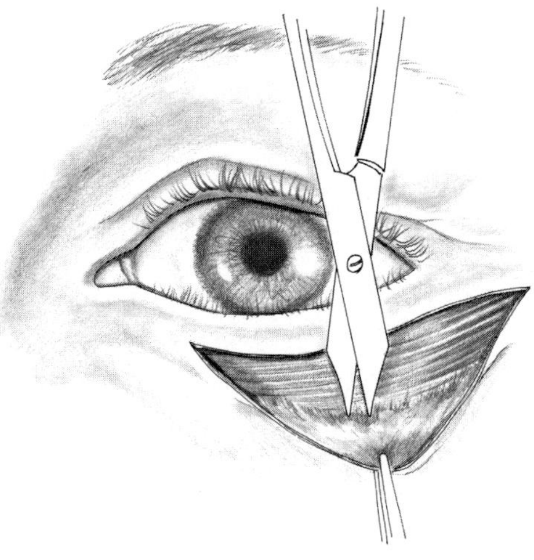

C, Skin dissected free from underlying orbicularis.

About 3 mm below the lash line, the orbicularis is incised parallel to the initial skin incision from its medial aspect to its temporal extremity. A strip of orbicularis muscle, which should be 7 to 10 mm wide to include the pretarsal and preseptal portions, is then prepared. A muscle hook is useful in grasping the muscle while the underlying fascia is dissected free (Plate 8-2, *D* and *E*).

At the temporal extremity of the dissection, the orbicularis strip is cut free (Plate 8-2, *F*). At this point the surgeon must decide if orbital fat should be excised. If so, after the septum has been opened with the spreading action of a hemostat or blunt scissors, the fat that is easily prolapsed is gently grasped with minimal traction and clamped. The fat is excised (Plate 8-2, *G*) and hemostasis is achieved with cautery before the fat is released. The septum is not closed with sutures. Lipolytic diathermy is used to further cauterize and retract the fat.

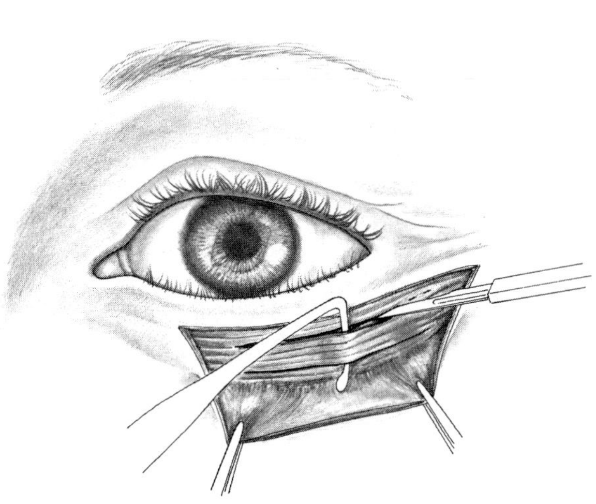

D, Strip of orbicularis (10 mm wide) dissected free.

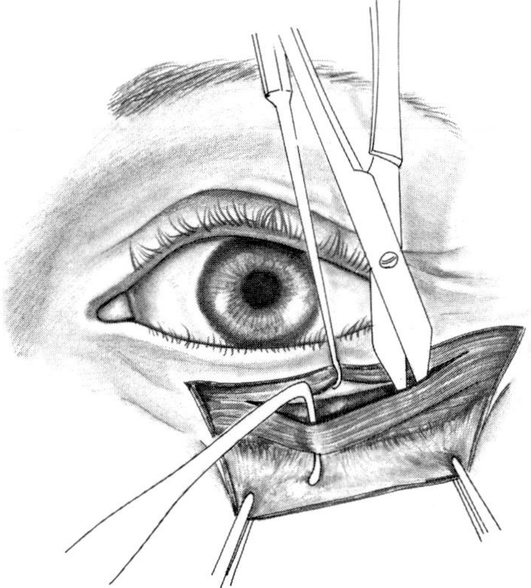

E, Orbicularis dissected free from underlying tissue.

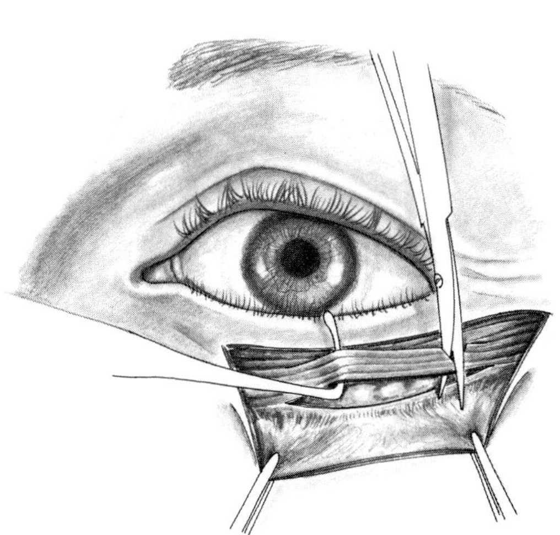

F, Temporal extremity of orbicularis strip released.

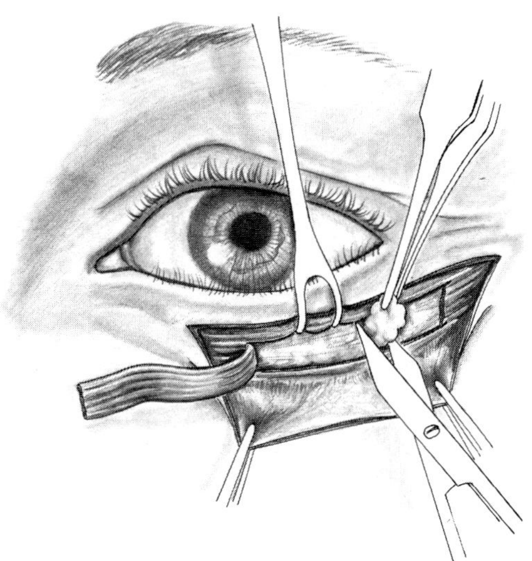

G, Excision of prolapsing orbital fat.

The temporal extremity of the strip is then grasped with a hemostat. On the temporal aspect of the inferior orbital rim, scissors are used to dissect down to periosteum (Plate 8-2, *H*). A double-armed 5-0 prolene suture is passed through the periosteum two times and passed through the temporal aspect of the orbicularis band (Plate 8-2, *I*). The tension of the band is adjusted as it is tied down to the periosteum. Excessive traction will cause deformity of the lid margin in the opposite direction. Two 5-0 Dexon sutures are placed to secure the strip in position (Plate 8-2, *J*). The overlying skin is then placed over the lid margin and excessive skin excised as in a lower-lid blepharoplasty. Interrupted 6-0 or mild chromic sutures are placed to close the incision (Plate 8-2, *K*). A light dressing is applied.

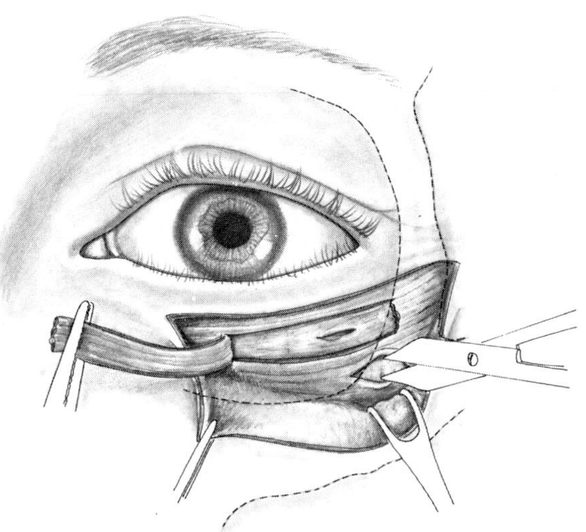

H, Dissection extended to level of periosteum of inferior orbital rim.

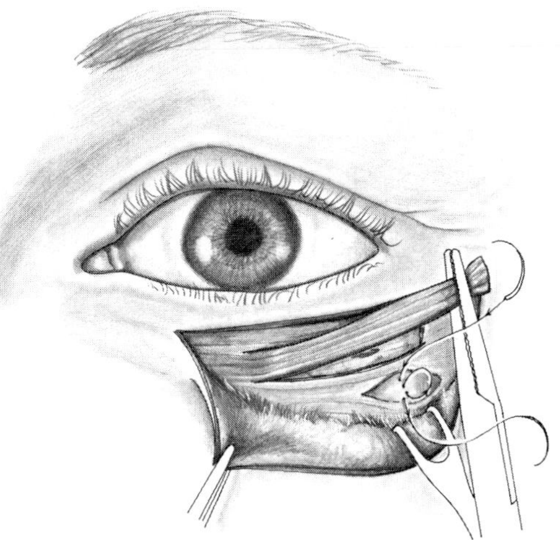

I, Temporal extremity of orbicularis band ready to be sutured to periosteum.

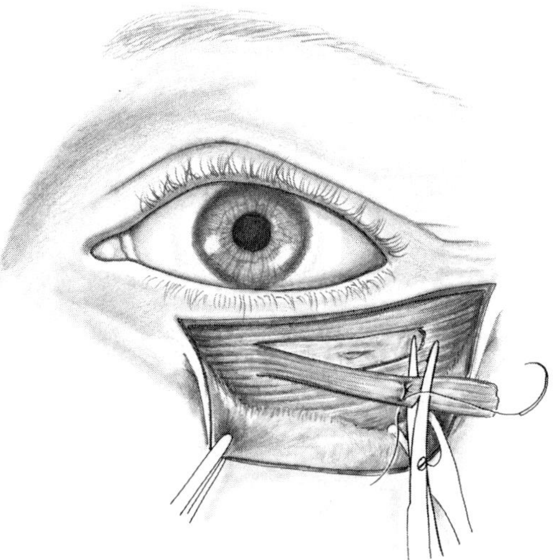

J, Tension of band adjusted and excess tissue excised.

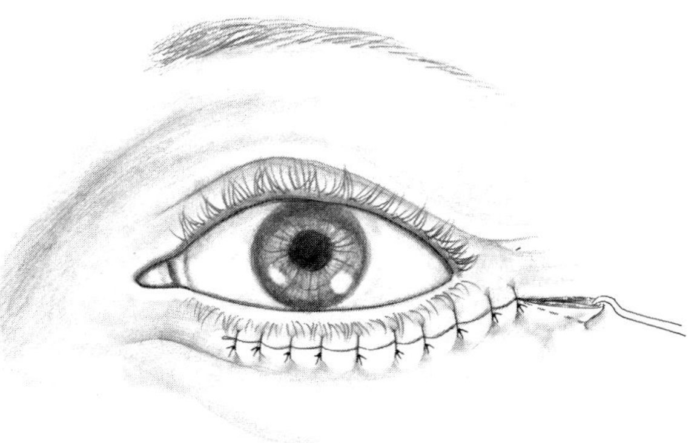

K, Redundant skin to be excised and skin layer closed.

Segmental cicatricial entropion of the upper lid may be corrected with a mucous membrane graft. The area of scarring may be excised with sharp dissection and covered with buccal mucosa. A 4-0 silk suture is placed through the skin and tarsus near the lid margin, and the eyelid is everted over a Desmarres retractor. The cicatricial area is excised, and the surrounding tissue is undermined and allowed to retract (Plate 8-3, *A*). The size of the mucosal graft is determined by direct measurement. The lower lip is everted over a clamp or with towel clips. The mucosa is ballooned away from the underlying tissue with the usual local anesthetic solution. Ideally, a Castroviejo mucotome is used to obtain a 0.5-mm-thick graft. Alternatively, a scalpel or iris scissors may be used to obtain the mucosal graft. Any attached subcutaneous tissue is carefully removed from the undersurface of the graft.

The graft is immediately layered on the recipient bed without moving away from the sterile field. It is sewn into position with several double-armed, 6-0 Vicryl sutures passed partial thickness through the graft's underside and then brought out through the skin surface and tied over rubber-band bolsters (Plate 8-3, *B*). The 4-0 silk traction suture placed at the beginning of the procedure is used to place the lid on stretch by taping the suture to the skin over the inferior orbital rim with Steri-Strips. A firm pressure dressing is placed over the lids. The traction suture and the Vicryl sutures are removed in 7 to 10 days.

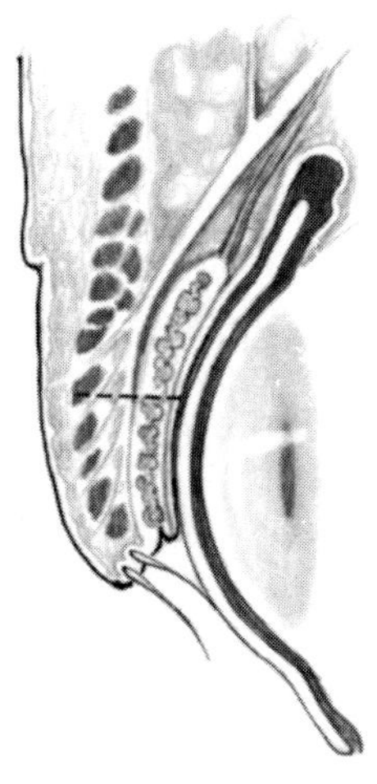

A, Upper-lid site designated and incised.

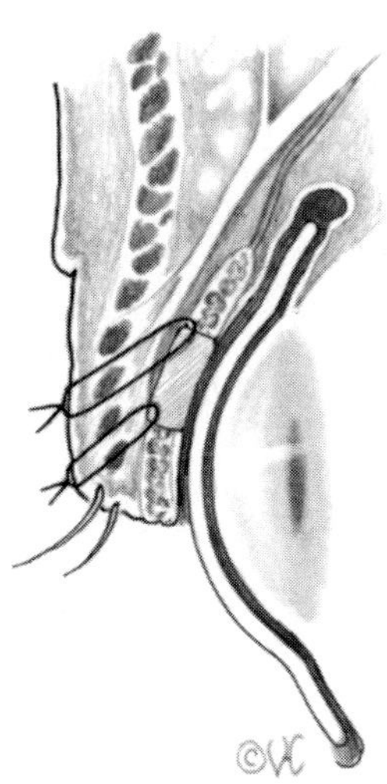

B, Donor graft sutured into recipient site.

For a more severe degree of cicatrization of the upper lid or in those cases in which a previous attempt at correction has failed, the procedure we prefer is through-and-through fracturing of the tarsus combined with external rotation of the lid margin. Often, there is complete shrinkage of all of the layers of the lid and a procedure affecting only internal or external layers of that lid will not be sufficient for correction.

The inwardly rotated lid is grasped on its external surface and outwardly rotated. About 4 mm above the lash line a marking pen is used to designate the line of incision from the medial to the temporal aspect of the lid, 2 to 3 mm beyond the area of lid malposition (Plate 8-4, *A*).

A razor knife is used to incise along the line down through the skin and into the orbicularis (Plate 8-4, *B*). A full-thickness penetration is not sought, because of the possibility of angling the incision and of damaging the marginal arterial arcade, which is present within 3 mm of the lid margin. The lid is everted and, with the lid margin in view, an incision at a similar distance is made through the tarsus and the conjunctiva (Plate 8-4, *C*).

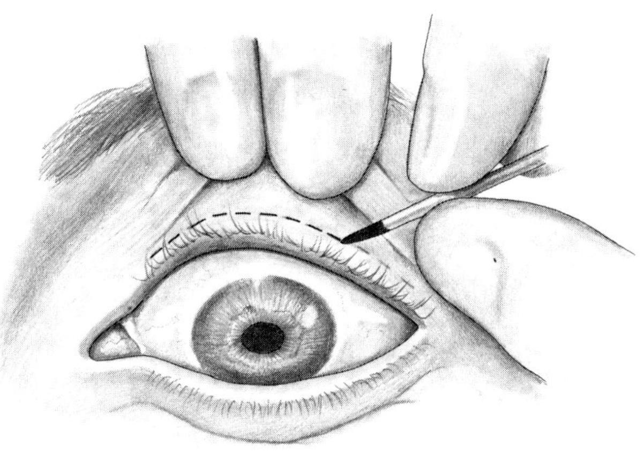

A, Inverted lid margin extra-rotated and line of incision marked.

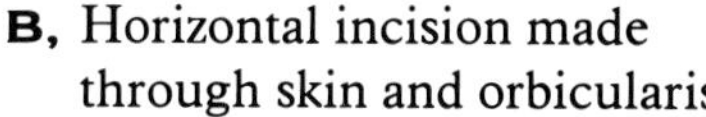
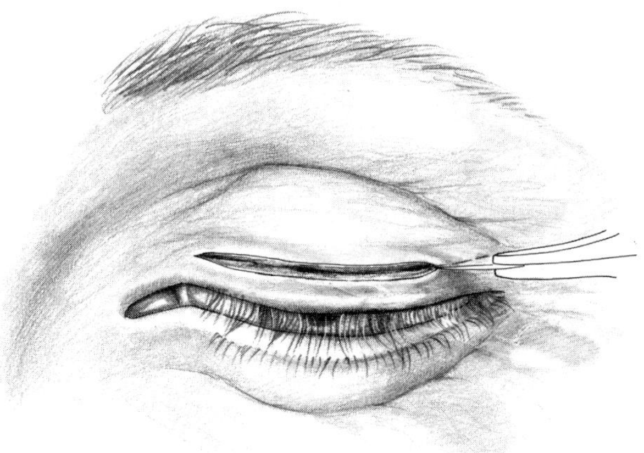

B, Horizontal incision made through skin and orbicularis.

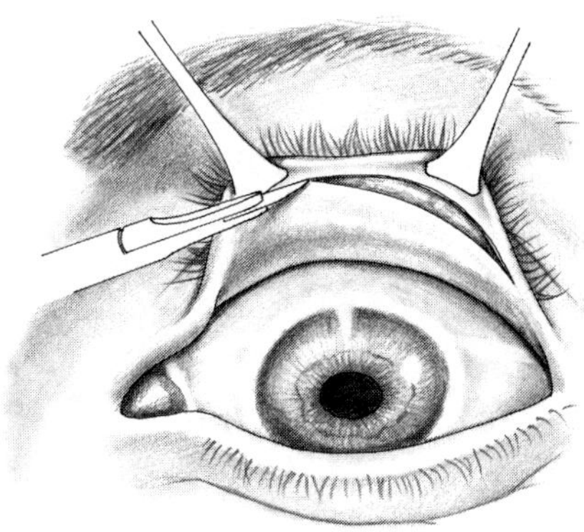

C, Upper lid everted and tarsus incised opposite skin incision.

With the lid in the normal position, iris scissors are used to complete the transverse blepharotomy incision (Plate 8-4, *D*). The lid margin having been freed, a 4-0 double-armed suture is passed centrally from the conjunctival side of the lid tissue, through the tarsus, and withdrawn from the middle lamella of the upper aspect of the wound (Plate 8-4, *E*). This double-armed suture is then passed through the lid margin bridge and withdrawn just above the lash line (Plate 8-4, *F*).

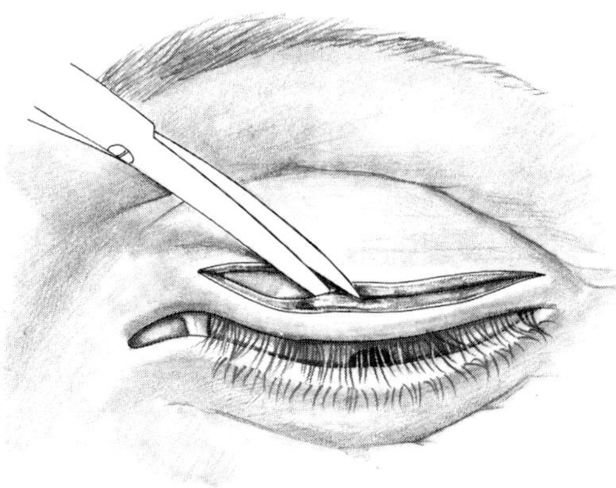

D, Scissors used to join two incisions.

E, Double-armed silk suture placed from conjunctival level outward.

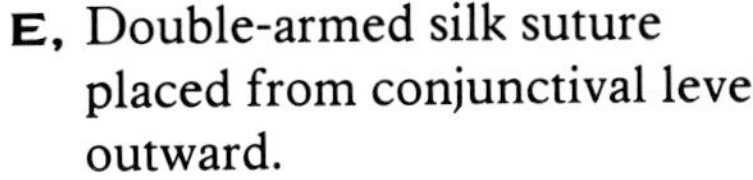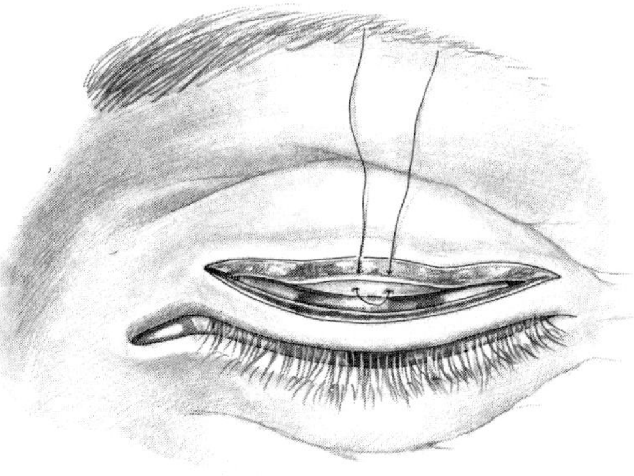

F, Suture brought through lid just above tarsus and out of lid margin above lash line.

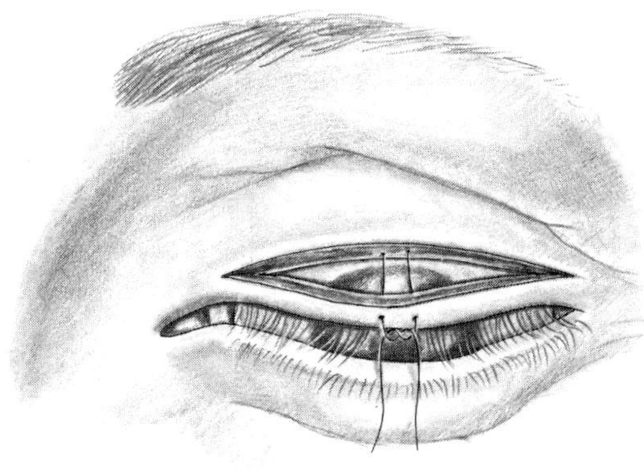

The inwardly turned upper lid margin has now been transversely incised and the marginal strip of lid externally rotated and secured into its new position (Plate 8-4, *G*). Approximately four of these 4-0 double-armed silk sutures are placed (Plate 8-4, *H*). These are tied sufficiently tight to ensure a slight overcorrection of the lid margin. These sutures can be tied over rubber-band bolsters.

The upper skin edge is closed with interrupted 6-0 mild chromic sutures, and a light dressing is applied. The mattress sutures are removed after 7 to 10 days.

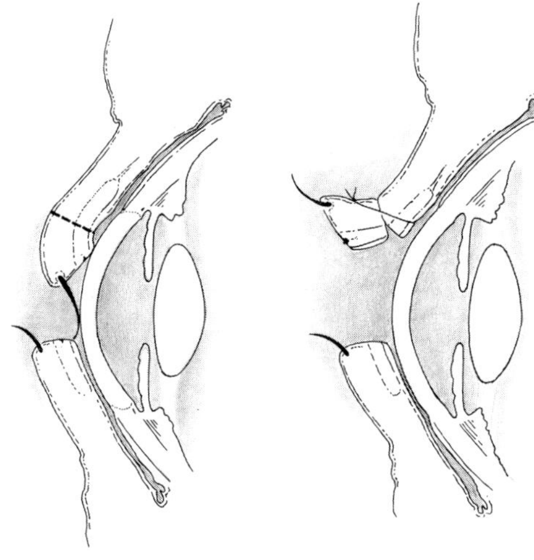

G, Sagittal view demonstrating entropic upper lid and placement of initial suture.

H, Lid in final position with several double-armed sutures in place and skin closed.

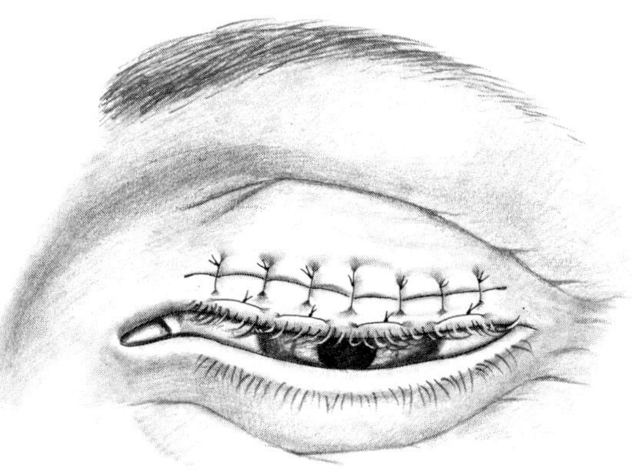

REATTACHMENT OF THE
LOWER-LID RETRACTORS

After the lid has been infiltrated with 2% lidocaine in 1:100,000 epinephrine, a marking pen is used to designate a subciliary incision 2 mm below the lash line (Plate 8-5, *A*). A razor knife is later used to incise the previously demarcated area. A skin-muscle flap is then dissected down almost to the inferior orbital rim (Plate 8-5, *B*).

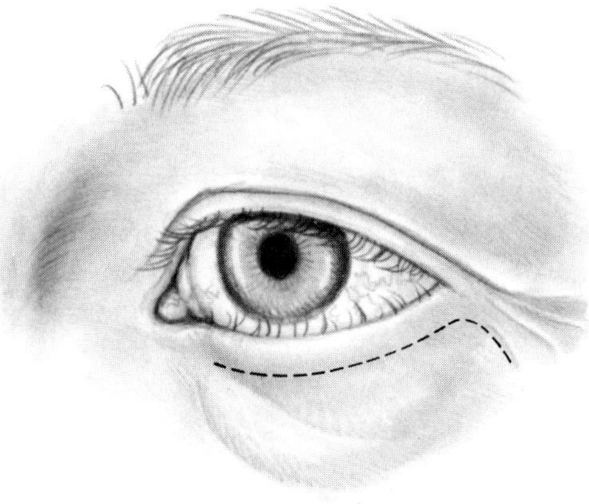

A, Inwardly rotated lower eyelid with subciliary incision marked.

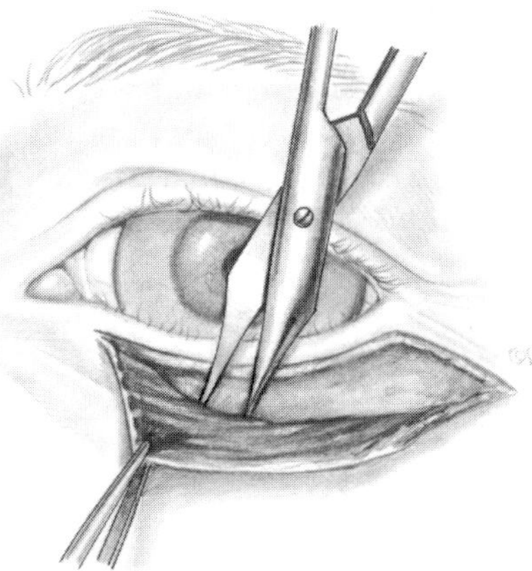

B, Incision made 2 mm below lash line and myocutaneous flap dissected.

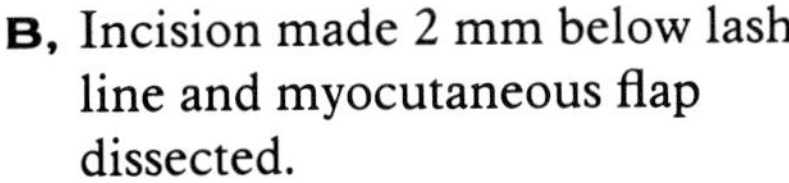

C, Pretarsal orbicularis removed and detached capsulopalpebral fascia shown.

D, Sagittal view demonstrating lid dissection and detached capsulopalpebral fascia.

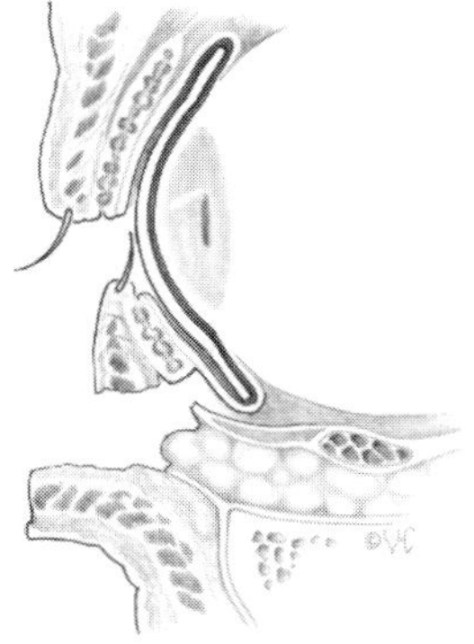

The flap is retracted with a Desmarres retractor and reflected anteriorly. Pretarsal orbicularis is excised from the inferior border of the tarsal plate (Plate 8-5, *C*). Hemostasis is achieved with thermal cautery. The patient is asked to repeatedly look upward toward the top of his head and then downward toward his feet while the surgeon observes the area just below the inferior border of the tarsus. A recurrent depression will be seen in this area with each downward glance. The most anterior aspect of the detached capsulopalpebral fascia will be found at this point (Plate 8-5, *D*). The depressed area is grasped with the Castroviejo forceps and pulled superiorly at a 45-degree angle to a plane parallel to the tarsus. The septum anterior to the capsulopalpebral fascia is dissected away to expose the dense, pearly white fascia. The patient is asked to look upward and downward again to confirm that the fascia has been dissected. The fascia will pull sharply out of forceps that gently grasp it. With the septum open, the fat pads are exposed. They are important landmarks, since the retractors are posterior to them. The fascia is reattached to the inferior border of the tarsus with several interrupted 5-0 Novafil sutures. These may be placed to include the skin incision and enhance the rotational effect or to not include the skin and thus obtain a less obvious incision (Plate 8-5, *E* to *H*). The skin incision is closed with interrupted 6-0 mild chromic sutures (Plate 8-5, *I*).

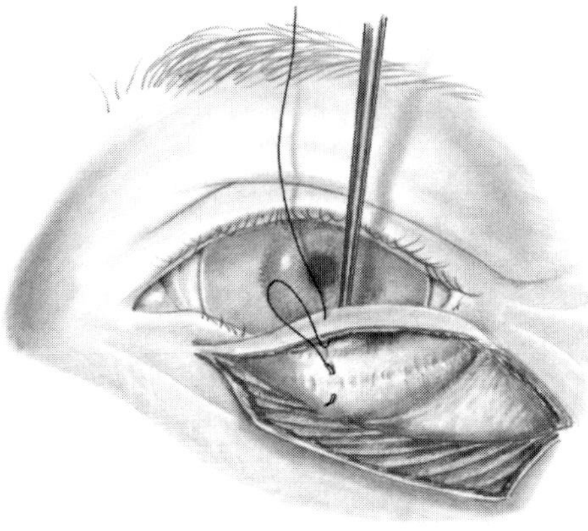

E, Needle passed through skin and inferior border of tarsus with 5-0 Novafil suture.

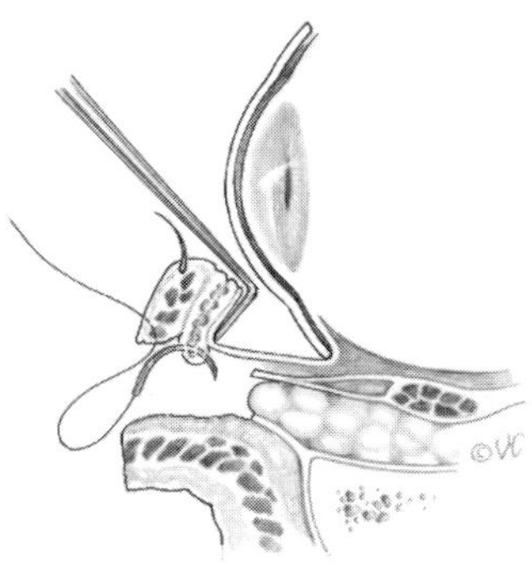

F, Sagittal view of needle passed through inferior border of tarsus.

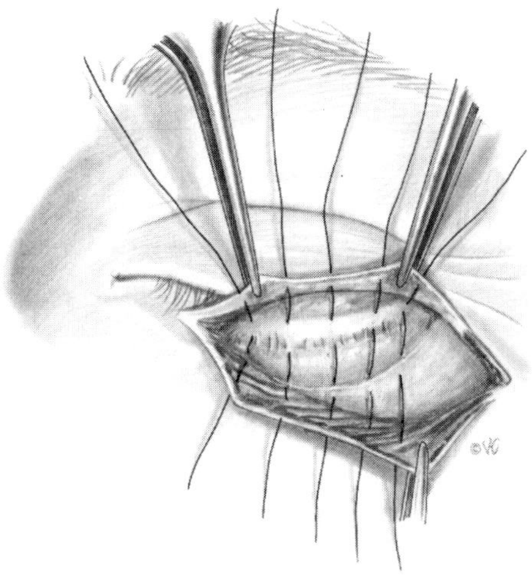

G, Multiple 5-0 Novafil sutures passed through inferior border of tarsus and detached capsulopalpebral fascia.

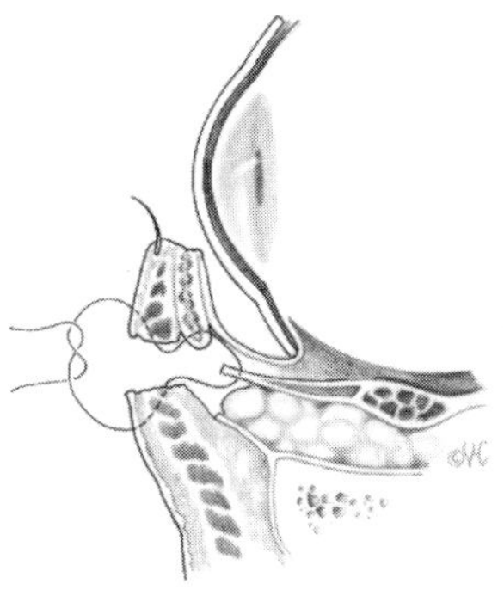

H, Sagittal view of final placement of 5-0 Novafil suture.

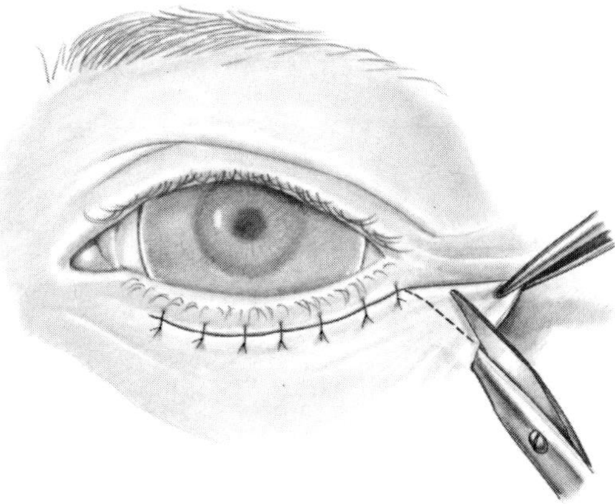

I, Final trimming of excess tissue.

ECTROPION REPAIR

Ectropion is the outward rotation of the lid margin. It can be cicatricial or noncicatricial. The noncicatricial type is an involutional process with gradual laxity of the lid combined with laxity of its supporting structures, the medial and lateral canthal tendons. Because of this laxity, there is an increase in the horizontal length of the lid. As time passes, a cicatrization of the lid tissues is produced within the lid, and thus a cicatricial component is added to the process. Cicatricial ectropion is a contracture of the anterior tissues of the lid. As time passes, this produces a horizontal lengthening of the lid. The excess horizontal length must be taken into account.

The repair of noncicatricial ectropion is performed by correcting the horizontal lengthening and laxity of the lid. To ascertain the degree of horizontal laxity, it is generally necessary to free the vertically shortened and fibrosed external layers of the lid from the inner lamellae. After these fibrotic tissues, the cicatricial element of the ectropion, have been separated from the remainder of the lid, one can better determine the true degree of laxity present. When the cicatricial component produces a shortage of external tissue, it is necessary to replace this tissue with a free skin graft or to employ one of the other procedures previously described.

Surgical repair of horizontal lid laxity (Plate 9-1, *A*) is best accomplished with a lateral tarsal strip. The lower lid and lateral canthal area are infiltrated with 2% lidocaine with 1:100,000 epinephrine. The lateral canthal area is the designated incision site (Plate 9-1, *B*). The lateral canthus is clamped with a small hemostat, and a lateral canthotomy is performed through the crushed tissue to the orbital rim (Plate 9-1, *C*). The lid is divided into anterior and posterior lamellae at the gray line, anterior to the tarsal plate (Plate 9-1, *D*). The estimated area of anterior lamella is excised. The lateral aspect of the lower lid is grasped, and a cantholysis is performed by severing the attachments between the tarsus and underlying tissues under direct visualization to minimize unnecessary dissection and hemorrhage. The completely freed lower lid is now pulled laterally enough to correct the lid laxity without causing the lower eyelid margin to drop. The position of the proposed new lateral canthus is again checked on the margin of the lower lid (Plate 9-1, *E*).

The lid margin is removed lateral to this mark with the razor knife. The posterior surface of the lid lateral to the mark is scraped with the razor knife. All tissue anterior and inferior to the tarsus and lateral to the mark is dissected away from the tarsus with iris scissors. Hemostasis is achieved with thermal cautery.

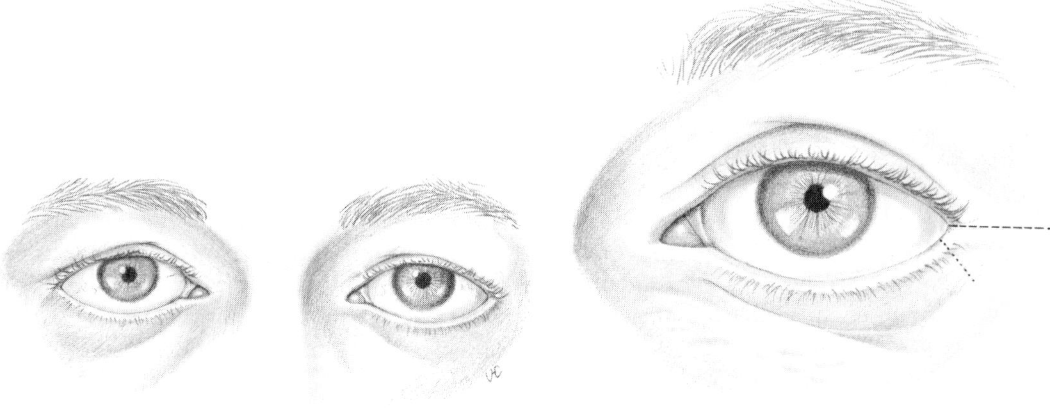

A, Bilateral lower-lid ectropion.

B, Lateral canthal area is the designated incision site (*long dashes*). Estimate of tarsal excision is shown (*short dashes*).

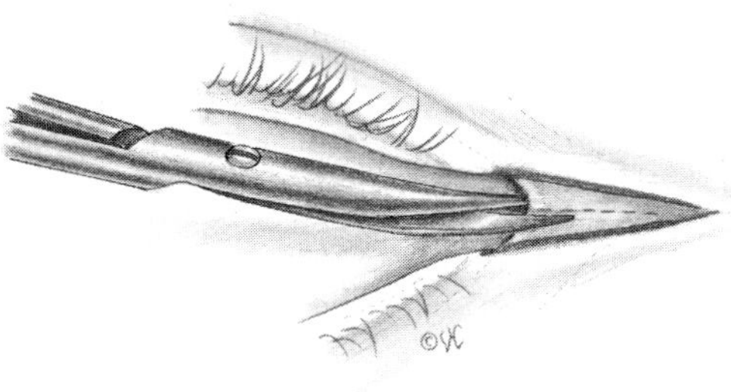

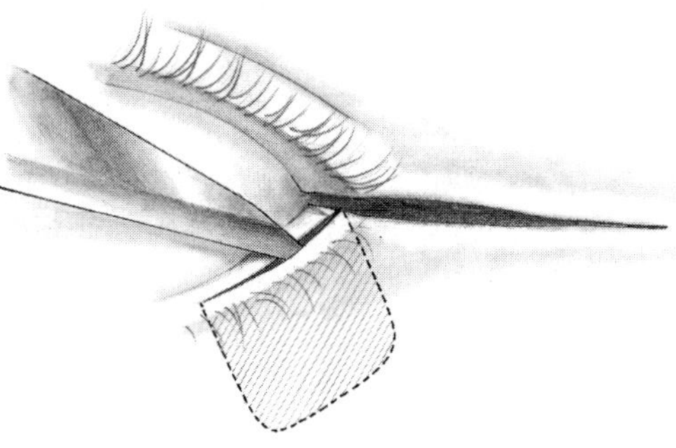

C, Lateral canthotomy performed, with incision carried to the orbital rim.

D, Lid divided at gray line, anterior to tarsal plate.

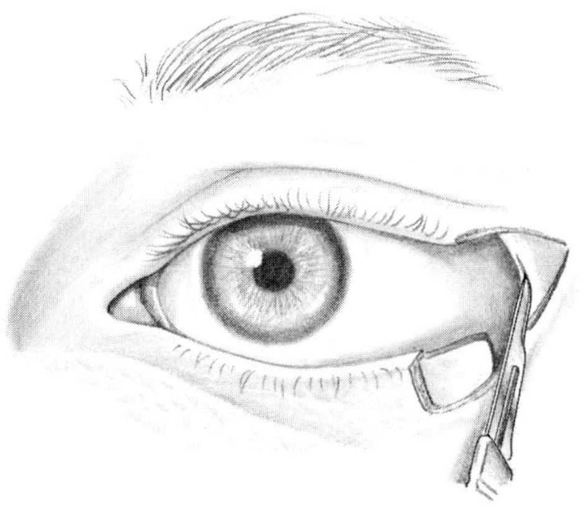

E, Inferior-crus cantholysis performed and lateral orbital rim incised.

Both needles of a double-armed 5-0 prolene suture with OPS-5 needles are passed anterior to posterior through the newly created tarsal tongue (Plate 9-1, *F, left*). The needles are passed through the tarsus near opposite edges to create as thick a bridge of tarsus as possible between suture. The white periosteum of the lateral orbital wall above the horizontal raphe has been exposed with a blade.

Each needle is grasped at its midpoint to ensure complete control during the periosteal suture pass. The needle is kept parallel to the axial plane. The needle tip is always directed away from the eye. The needle tip is positioned on top of the lateral orbital rim over the exposed periosteum at the proposed point of attachment. The needle tip is pulled medially while a subtle pressure is maintained against the orbital rim. The needle enters the periosteum just inside of the orbital rim, passing underneath it, and exits it just outside the orbital rim. Both needles are passed in similar fashion, with their orientation to each other being maintained, to create a horizontal mattress suture between the tarsus and the orbital periosteum (Plate 9-1, *F, right*).

Three throws are placed in the suture, and it is slowly tightened while the surgeon observes the lower eyelid as it is pulled laterally. The lid is pulled snugly toward the lateral canthus, but not to the point of causing the lateral lid to stand off from the globe or to the point of causing the lid level to drop relative to the lower limbus. The usual goal is to create a gentle upward curve to the lower lid, resulting in the lateral canthus being 2 mm superior to the medial canthus. The tarsus and superior crus of the lateral canthal tendon are sutured with 5-0 Vicryl.

The lateral canthus is re-formed by passing 6-0 mild chromic suture through the raw edge of the lower lid and out through the posterior lash line 2 mm from the lateral edge. The suture is then passed into the middle of the lash line of the superior lid 2 mm from the lateral edge and out through the raw edge. The knot is tied firmly with several throws, and the suture is cut 3 mm from the knot (Plate 9-1, *G*). The subcutaneous layer is then closed. The myocutaneous flap is draped over the incision, and any excess tissue is removed in the manner described in the blepharoplasty section. The incision is closed with 6-0 mild chromic suture (Plate 9-1, *H*). The eye is firmly patched until the following morning.

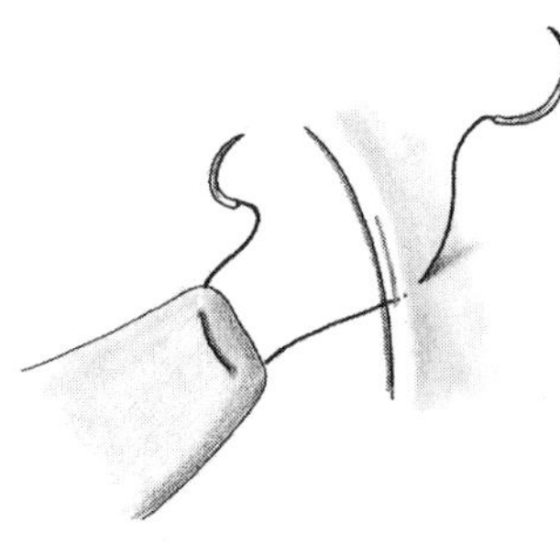 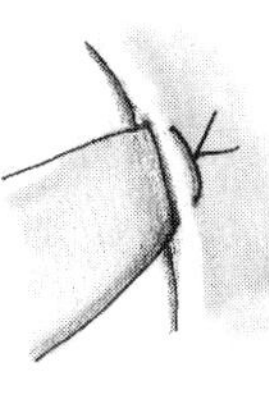

F, 5-0 prolene suture used to attach lateral tarsal strip to lateral orbital rim.

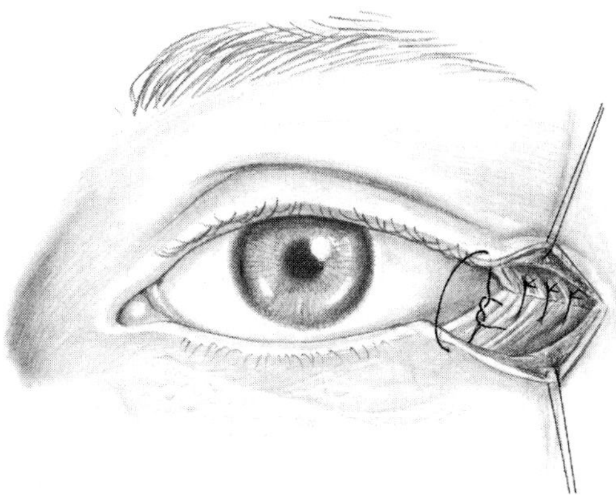

G, Lateral canthal angle is re-formed and subcutaneous tissue sutured.

H, Incision site sutured.

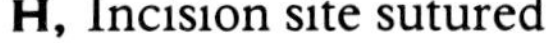 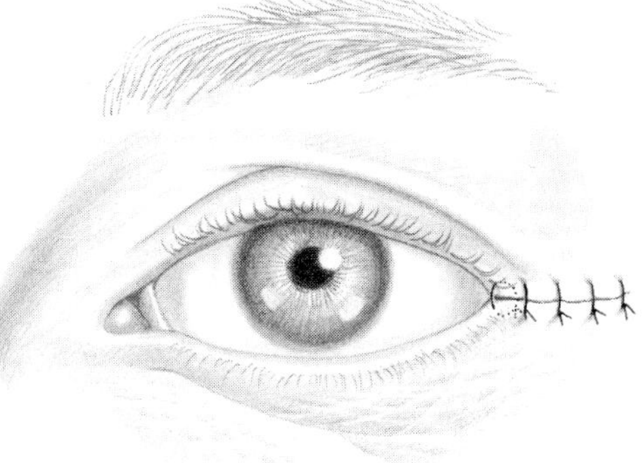

For the correction of an involutional ectropion with a lateral or complete eversion of the lid margin, we generally perform a full-thickness horizontal shortening of the lid under a blepharoplasty-type skin flap.

After a protective contact shell has been placed over the globe, a methylene blue marking pencil is used to designate an area for a subciliary incision about 2 mm below the lash line and extending from just below the punctum to the temporal smile fold at the lateral canthus (Plate 9-2, *A*). The lid is then anesthetized with 2% lidocaine with 1:100,000 epinephrine to provide lid akinesia and hydraulic dissection.

After the skin is incised along the demarcated area with a razor knife, the skin is separated from the underlying orbicularis down to the level of the inferior orbital rim. The dissection is slowly and carefully performed so as not to macerate the orbicularis fibers. The hydraulic dissection achieved with the local injection of anesthetic usually facilitates this maneuver, although it is a difficult technique to master. With the skin adequately dissected from the orbicularis, the lid is now freely movable and the full degree of laxity is demonstrable (Plate 9-2, *B*).

About one-fourth the distance from the lateral canthus, a full-thickness incision is made through the lid margin to about 2 mm below the tarsus. The incision then turns medially to form half of a pentagon. The lateral aspect of the lid is overlapped by the remainder of the lid, and the amount of tissue that needs to be excised is ascertained. The pentagonal wedge is then completed in the desired area. The second incision should be made parallel to the first so that lid closure results in a uniform lid margin with no notching of the lid.

The lid margin is closed by the three-suture technique, with the tarsal layer closed in this case to include overlying orbicularis. Absorbable 5-0 sutures are used for the closure (Plate 9-2, *C*).

The skin flap is drawn up and gently pulled laterally; any redundant skin is excised (Plate 9-2, *D*). If the cicatricial component has been extensive, the external layer of the lid may have to be replaced. The incision is then closed with interrupted or continuous 6-0 silk sutures (Plate 9-2, *E*).

A light dressing is applied to the wound. This is generally removed on the final postoperative day. The skin sutures are removed after 4 days and the marginal sutures 3 to 6 days later.

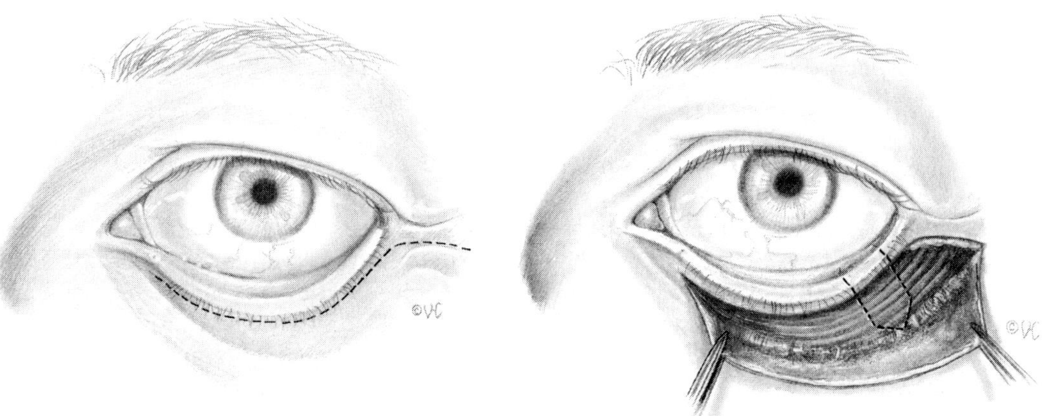

A, Subciliary incision outlined. Note lateral extension of line.

B, Skin dissected free from orbicularis and fibrotic tissue; pentagon-shaped excision outlined.

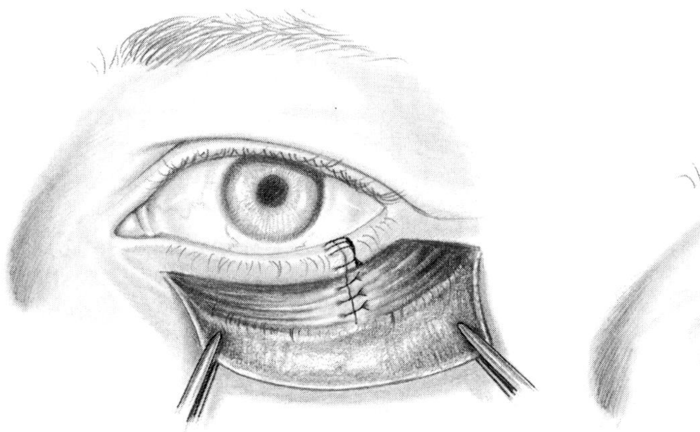

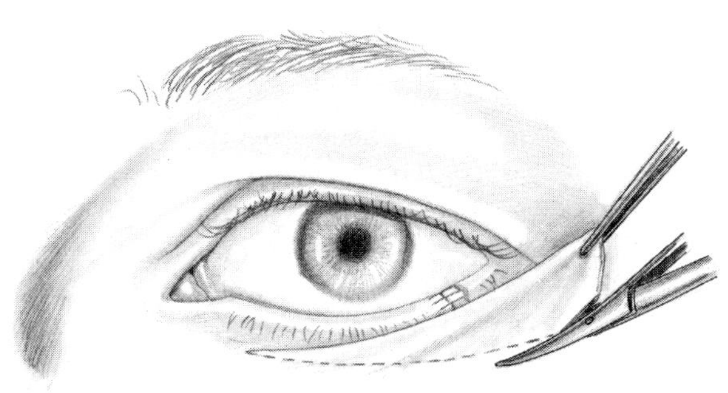

C, Lid horizontally shortened and closed with three-suture technique.

D, Redundant skin excised.

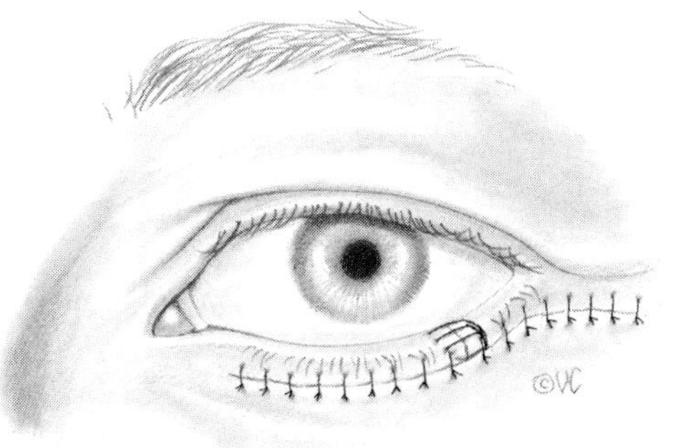

E, Closure with interrupted sutures.

Cicatricial ectropion is caused by vertical shortening of the anterior lamellae of the eyelid (Plate 9-3, *A*). Its correction usually requires lysis and excision of the fibrotic tissue and a free skin graft to allow the lid to return to a normal position. An ancillary lateral tarsal strip procedure is sometimes required to provide additional support for a severely affected lower lid.

A 4-0 silk traction suture is placed through the tarsus at the lid margin. A subciliary skin incision is made with a razor knife from just below the punctum laterally to the canthal angle and into a smile crease. The cicatricial tissue is dissected free with curved iris scissors and excised (Plate 9-3, *B*). Underlying vertically oriented fibrotic bands of scar tissue are sought and lysed if found (Plate 9-3, *C*). The lid position is now checked with the patient upright, and dissection is continued until the lid position is appropriate. A tarsal strip procedure may be done at this stage to correct a horizontal laxity that is only apparent after the cicatricial tissue has been removed. Thermal cautery is kept to a minimum to preserve a good vascular bed for the skin graft. Hemostasis is best achieved with gentle pressure and charged collagen products.

A donor site is selected for the skin graft and prepared in the usual fashion, as previously discussed. In most cases, a full-thickness skin graft is preferred. All subcutaneous tissue should be removed by placing the graft epidermis-side-down on a gloved finger and gently trimming away the fatty-appearing tissue. The graft is sutured into the recipient bed with interrupted 6-0 mild chromic suture (Plate 9-3, *D*). Several full-thickness fenestrations are placed in the graft to minimize postoperative fluid accumulation. The graft should always be held over the sterile field.

The original silk suture is used to place the lid on stretch. Several interrupted 6-0 mild chromic sutures to hold the bolster are placed 3 to 5 mm away from the graft margin. The graft is covered with antibiotic ointment. A single, moist Telfa dressing is layered over the graft and ointment to minimize adhesion between the bolster and the skin graft. A moist piece of cotton is placed over the Telfa to provide rigidity to the bolster. The 6-0 mild chromic suture is tied over the moist cotton, which will stiffen as it dries.

The donor site is now closed. The bolster and traction suture should stay in place for 5 to 7 days. Because the bolster is attached with mild chromic sutures placed away from the graft edge, their complete removal is not critical and they do not disturb the graft.

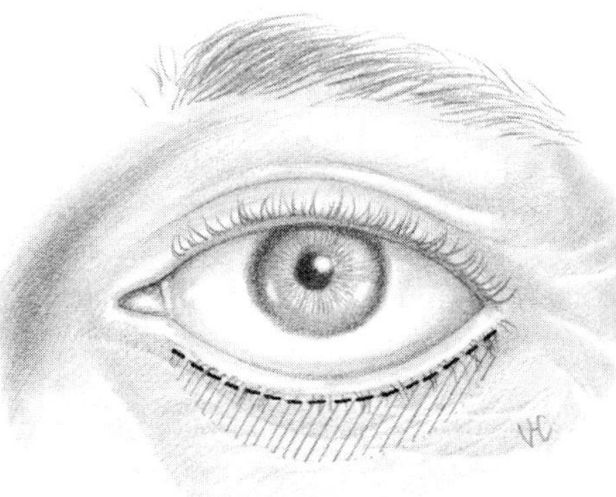

A, Vertical shortening of lower lid with scarring.

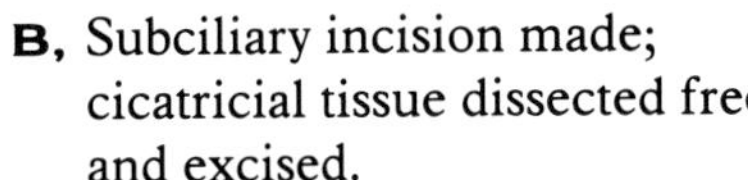

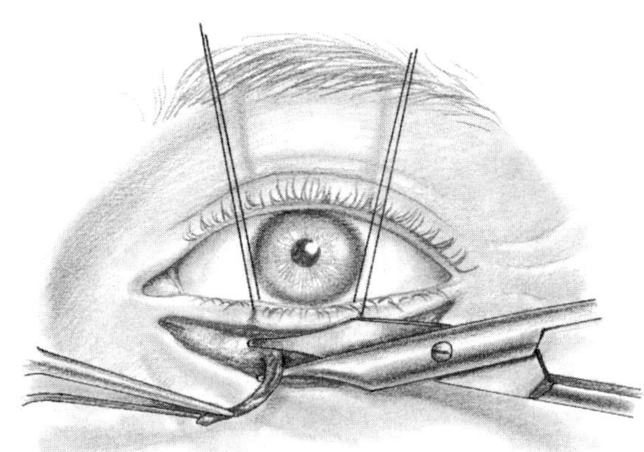

B, Subciliary incision made; cicatricial tissue dissected free and excised.

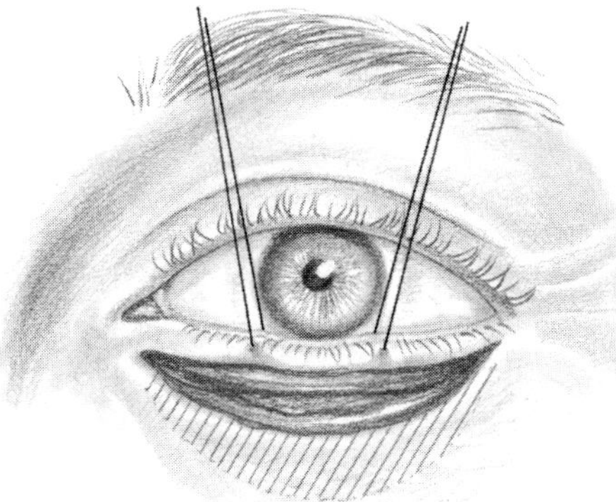

C, Vertical fibrotic bands lysed. Recipient bed ready for graft

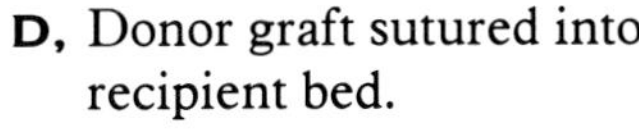

D, Donor graft sutured into recipient bed.

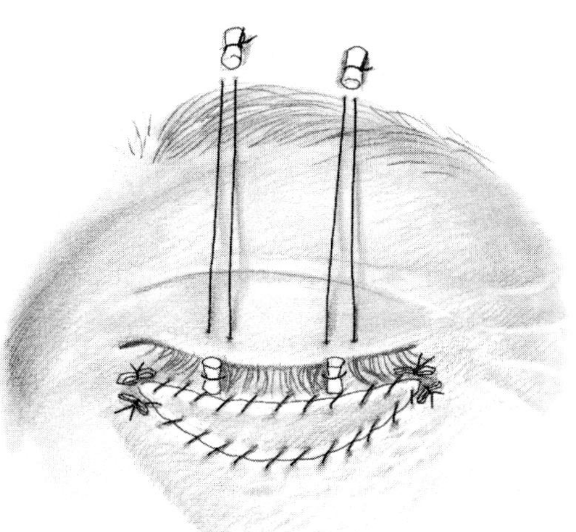

The lazy-T correction is useful for repairing an ectropion of the lower lid associated with frank punctal eversion, but not a distinct weakness of the medial canthal tendon. A V-shaped wedge is excised from the lid to correct the horizontal lengthening that may be present, while at the same time a horizontal incision through the conjunctiva and tarsus is used to correct the eversion of the lid (Plate 9-4, *A*). Although other techniques such as internal cautery of the lid and a horizontal excision of tarsoconjunctival tissue used alone have been advocated, we have found these to be associated with complications (the former) or insufficient to correct the underlying pathophysiology of the defect (the latter). A lateral tarsal strip procedure is another good choice in these situations.

Forceps are used to evert the lower lid. It may also be helpful to support the lid with a lid plate during the first part of the procedure. A probe is then inserted into the canaliculus to locate its horizontal level in the lid. Approximately 7 mm below the punctum an incision is made with a razor knife through conjunctiva and tarsus. The incision should be about 1 to 1½ cm in length, with the medial aspect of the incision extending slightly beyond the punctum (Plate 9-4, *B*).

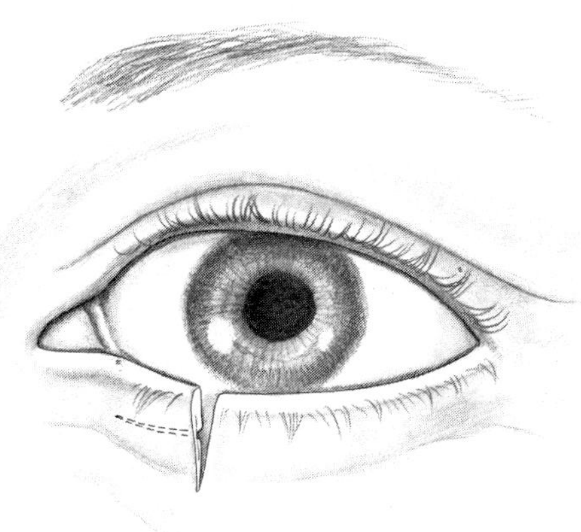

A, Combined horizontal and vertical shortening to produce lazy T.

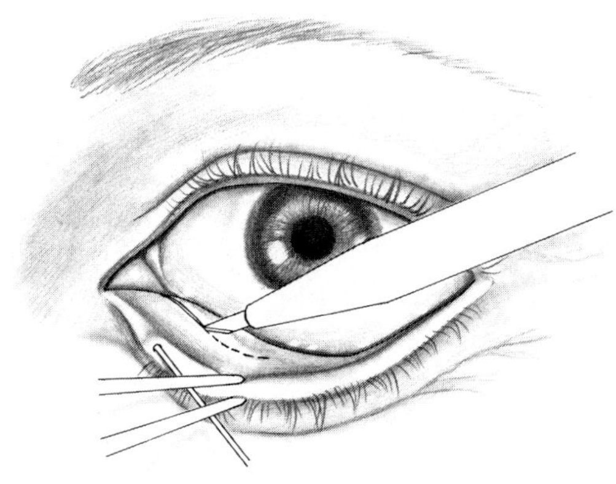

B, Initial incision through conjunctiva and tarsus.

Scissors are then used to undermine the inferior edge of the wound. This undermining should extend for about 3 to 5 mm (Plate 9-4, *C* and *D*). With sufficient undermining, the inferior aspect of the incision can overlap the superior portion of the wound. It is useful to employ two pairs of forceps, each grasping an alternate end of the wound and thus facilitating the overlapping (Plate 9-4, *E* and *F*). The inferior wound edge is gently dissected, and the correct lid position is determined. The entire area that has been undermined is excised so that the lid will be held in the position into which it is sutured (Plate *9-4G*).

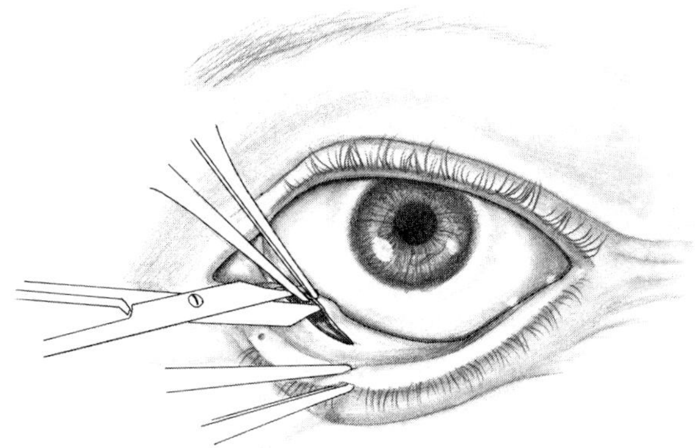

C, Inferior border of incision undermined.

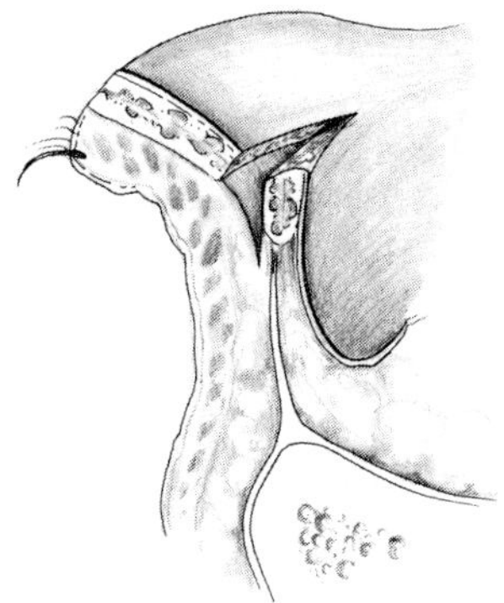

D, Cross section to illustrate incision.

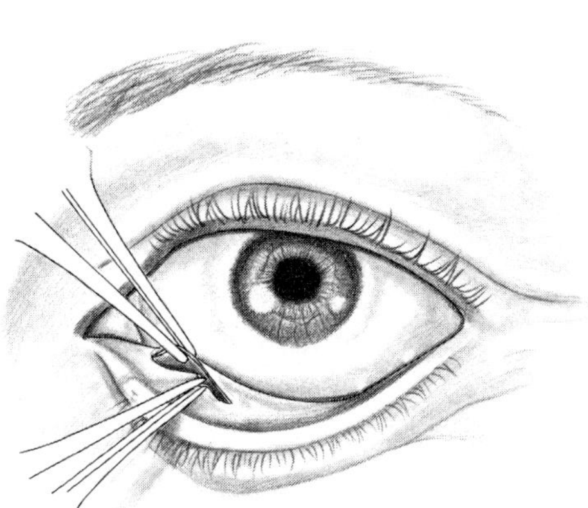

E, Inferior aspect of wound overlapped.

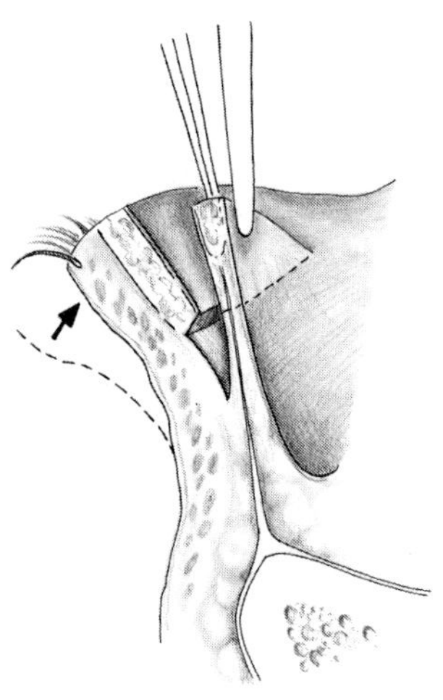

F, Cross section to illustrate overlapping.

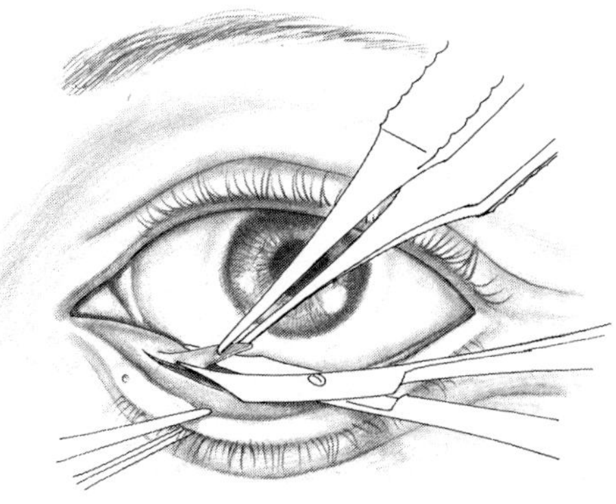

G, Excess tissue resected.

The horizontal lid laxity is corrected by making a full-thickness vertical incision of the lid 3 mm lateral to the punctum down to the lower fornix (Plate 9-4, *H*). With the surgeon using the double-armed forceps technique, the two edges of the incision are overlapped and the area to be excised is determined (Plate 9-4, *I* and *J*). The resection is sufficient to correct the horizontal laxity and place the lid in correct apposition with the globe. The resection takes a triangular wedge shape in the lid, which can be closed by the three-suture technique (Plate 9-4, *K*).

For closure of the horizontal tarsoconjunctival incision, we prefer 7-0 chromic catgut sutures. These are placed in an interrupted fashion and the knots pulled into the conjunctiva as much as possible. These generally cause no irritation. A pressure patch is applied until the following morning.

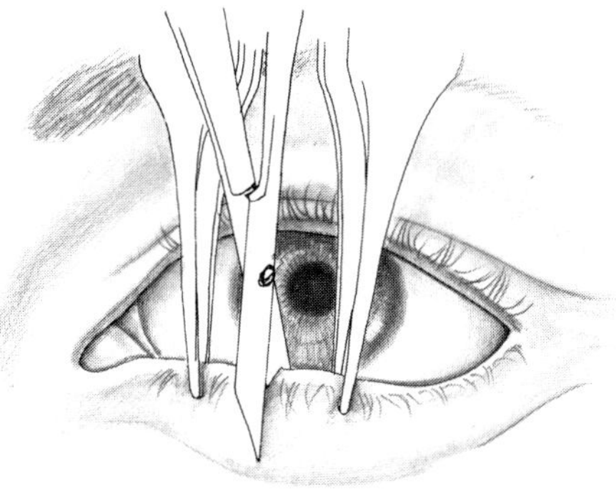

H, Full-thickness incision through lid margin.

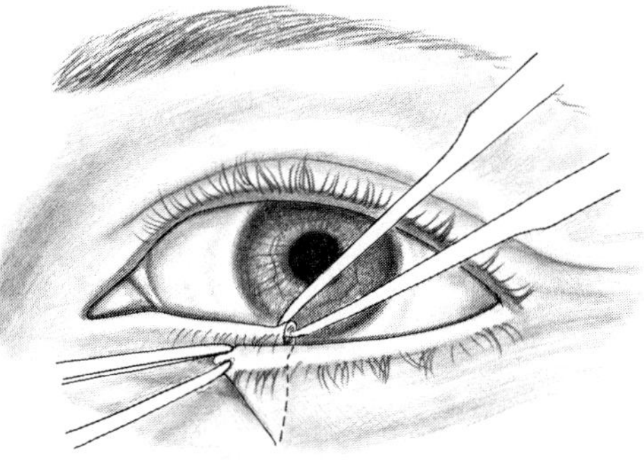

I, Lid margin overlapped and amount to be resected outlined.

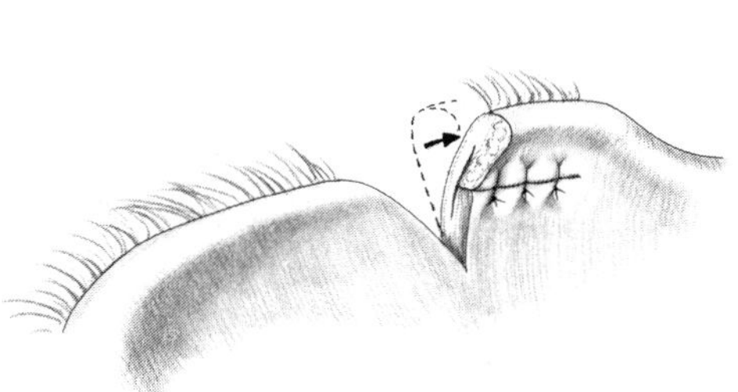

J, Inner aspect of lid to illustrate excessive lid tissue excised and tarsoconjunctival wound closed.

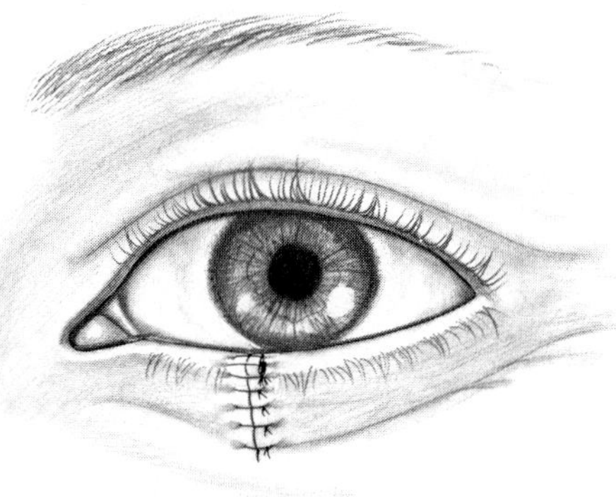

K, Closure of lid margin with three-suture technique.

COSMETIC BLEPHAROPLASTY

Dermatochalasis is an excess of skin in the upper or lower lids. It is commonly seen in the middle-aged and elderly. Excessive skin overhanging the supratarsal crease can override the lashes and lid margin of the upper lid, while in the lower lid it can cause excessive bagging. This condition may be associated with allergy, infection, or metabolic disturbances. It should be differentiated from blepharochalasis, which is a hereditary condition affecting young people, especially young adult women. The lid tissues are atrophied, causing skin redundancy and herniation of fat through the orbital upper-lid septum.

The procedures for correction of excessive lid skin and muscle are no longer reserved for cases with obstructive or fatigue symptoms. The current emphasis on youth has created an increasing need for the ophthalmologist to be familiar with these techniques.

Preoperatively a complete ophthalmologic evaluation of the patient should be performed. Photographic documentation is essential. Asymmetries of facial contour should be pointed out to the patient before surgery. A Schirmer test should be performed, since a mild overcorrection could cause a dry eye. Systemic causes of lid swelling, such as renal or thyroid disorders, should be kept in mind.

A marking pen is used to designate an area at or just (1 mm) above the supratarsal crease. Fixation forceps with the lower blade placed along the demarcated line are used to grasp the redundant lid skin. The skin is elevated, and the superior margin of the skin to be excised is marked (Plate 10-1, A). The incision size is limited by two factors: none of the thicker brow skin is excised, and sufficient lid skin must remain to avoid lid retraction. The fixation forceps are moved from the temporal aspect of the lid to the medial aspect, and each section is marked individually.

The redundant skin is ballooned away from orbicularis by injecting local anesthetic solution with epinephrine. The upper lid skin is stretched, and the incision is made with a razor knife. The incision is made into the orbicularis; it does not penetrate the septum (Plate 10-1, B). The skin and muscle between the incisions are removed with curved iris scissors while the area is continually blotted to maintain good visualization of the developing wound (Plate 10-1, C). Hemostasis is achieved with thermal cautery after the skin and muscle have been completely excised. The skin and muscle are kept sterile until the end of the procedure to allow repair of any possible overcorrection.

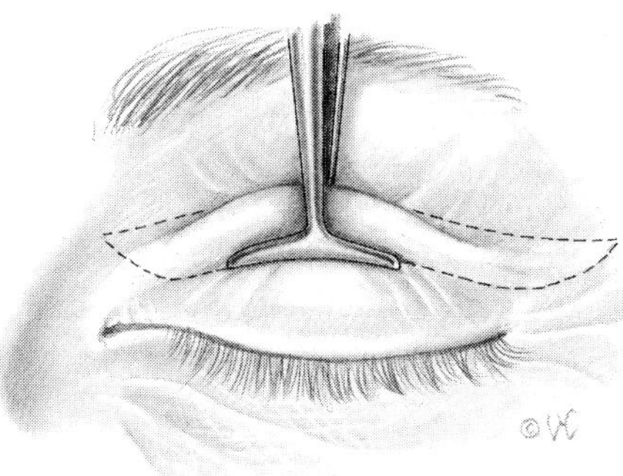

A, Forceps used to outline skin to be excised.

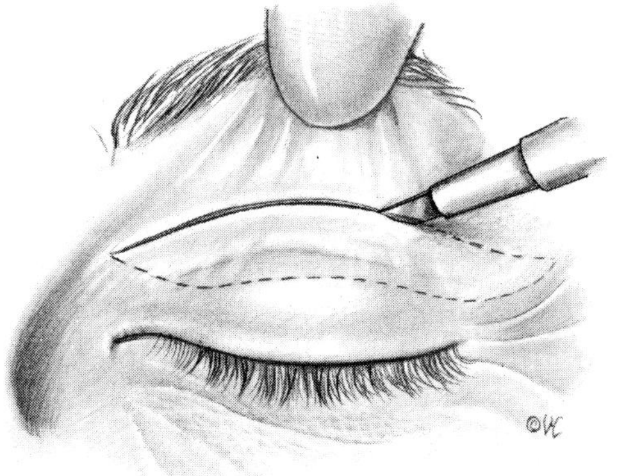

B, Razor knife used for incision.

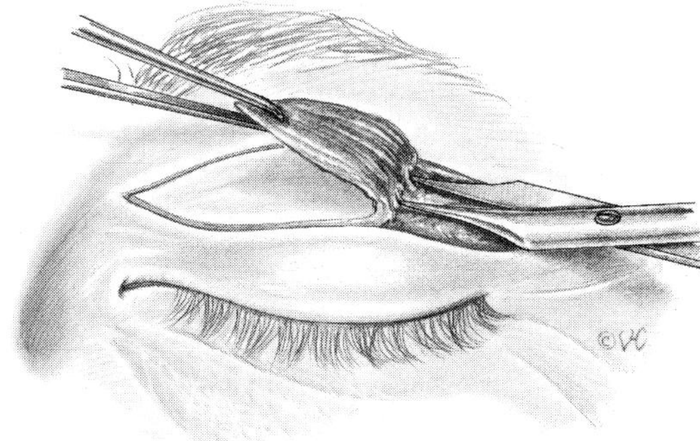

C, Scissors used to remove skin and orbicularis.

The orbital septum is opened in the area of desired orbital fat excision by tenting it anteriorly with forceps and removing a horizontal strip (Plate 10-1, *D*). The surgeon carefully avoids placing any instrument into the orbital fat without direct visualization to control its effects. The fat is brought anterior to the septum by injecting it with 1% lidocaine and by gentle digital pressure on the globe (Plate 10-1, *E* and *F*). The direct injection of lidocaine also greatly decreases the amount of sedation required for fat excision, the most painful part of the procedure.

After the fat is brought anterior to the orbital septum, it is clamped with a hemostat. The hemostat is supported at all times to avoid traction on the deep orbital vessels and possible deep orbital hemorrhage. The fat anterior to the hemostat is cut with scissors or cautery (Plate 10-1, *G*). The residual fat is vigorously cauterized prior to being released. The fat is grasped with forceps and is then released from the hemostat while the surgeon observes it for any bleeding. Bleeding from the fat is treated by clamping the fat more posterior than the bleeding point and repeating the steps above. After the desired amount of fat has been removed, the face of the remaining fat is treated with lipolytic diathermy to further retract the fat and minimize the risk of late bleeding.

The skin is closed with interrupted 6-0 mild chromic sutures attaching skin edge to skin edge. Continuous running sutures, 6-0 mild chromic or a nonabsorbable material, are also useful, but require more skill in their placement. Subcuticular sutures give an excellent cosmetic result, but are very difficult to remove, even with a center loop (Plate 10-1, *H*).

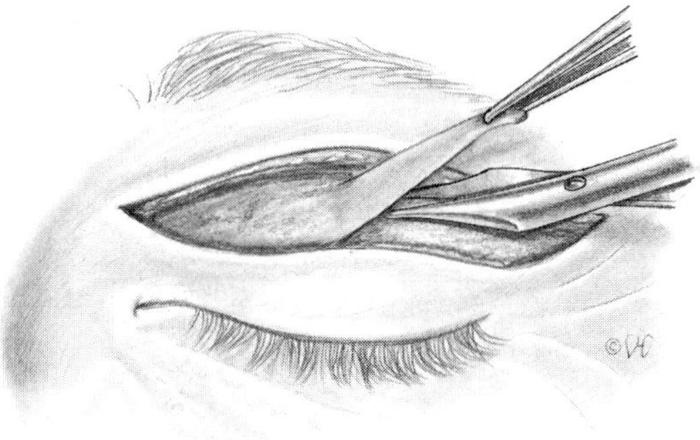

D, Orbital septum opened widely.

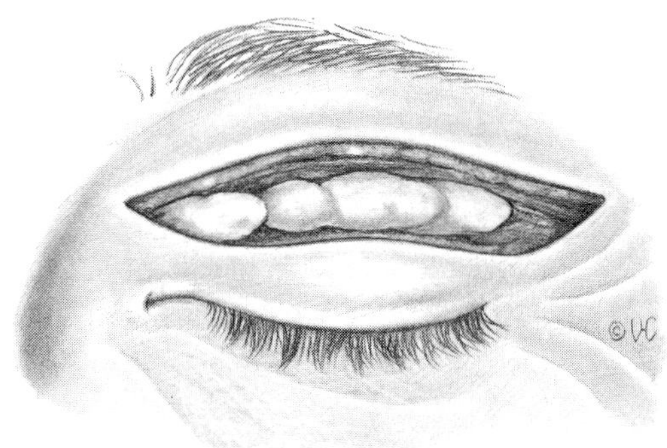

E, Upper-lid fat pads exposed. Remember, there is no lateral fat pad.

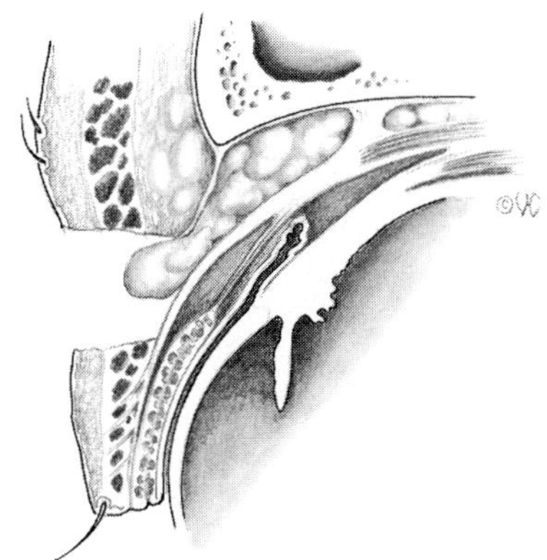

F, Sagittal view of orbital fat.

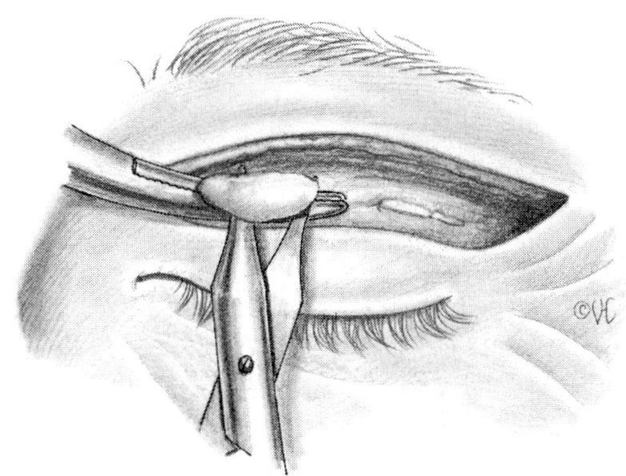

G, Fat pads excised.

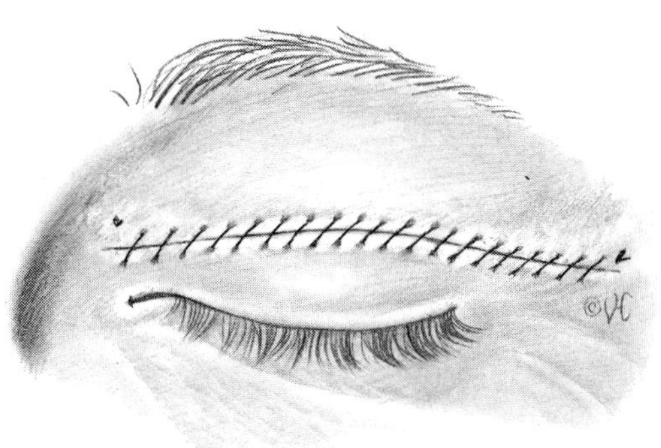

H, Continuous suture used to close the incision.

Following the closure of the upper lid, the marking pen is used to create a line 2 mm below the lashes of the lower lid from just below the punctum to the temporal smile crease, remaining at least 5 mm from the upper incision at this point to prevent webbing (Plate 10-2, *A*). After the injection of the local anesthetic, the blade is used to incise the lateral aspect of the previously demarcated area. The surgeon uses iris scissors or a hemostat to separate the skin from the orbicularis, taking care not to macerate the underlying orbicularis, which may cause postoperative wadding and unsightly bulges in the lid. The incision is then carried across the demarcated area. The dissection is carried to the level of the inferior orbital rim (Plate 10-2, *B*). Fat is removed in the fashion described for the upper lid (Plate 10-2, *C* to *F*).

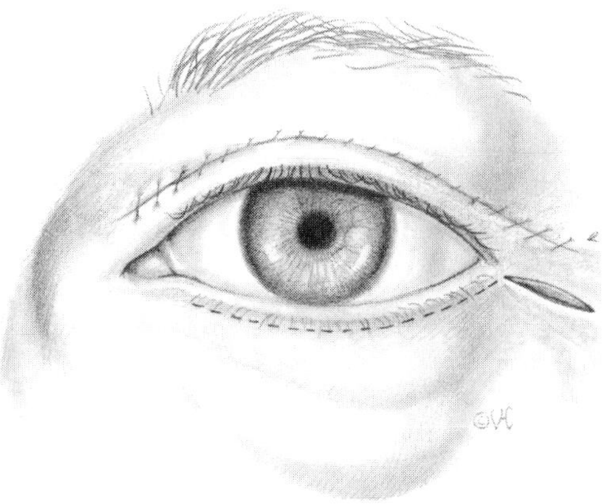

A, Lower lid marked 2 mm below lash line.

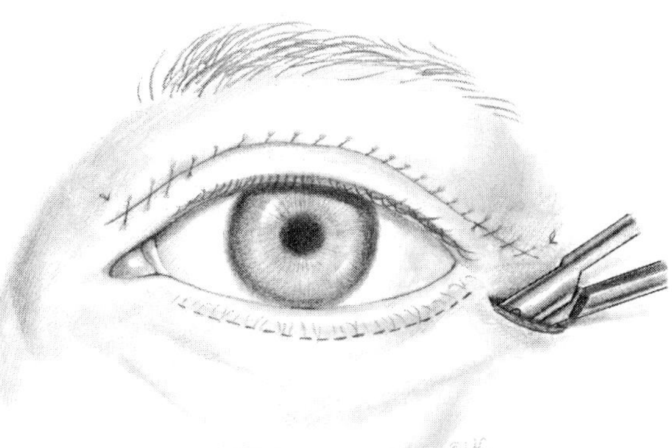

B, Blunt dissection used after initial incision is made.

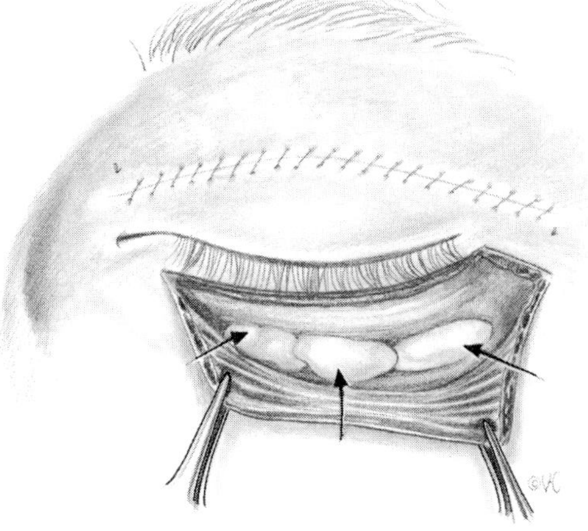

C, Septum removed and three lower-lid fat pads exposed.

D, Fat gently prolapsed.

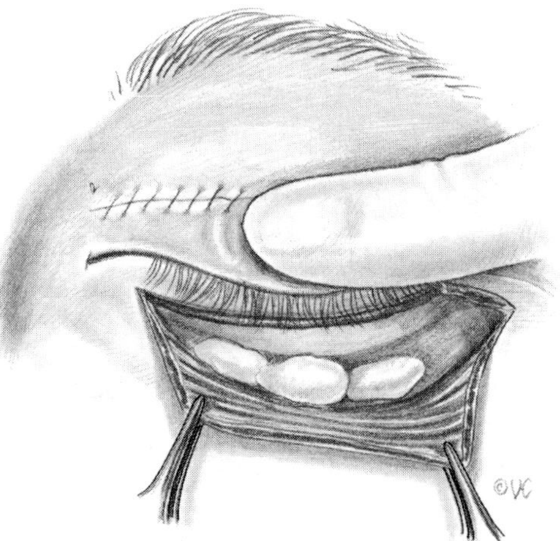

With care taken to release the surgical drape so the cheek position will not be artificially elevated, the globe is gently depressed. The amount of skin overlapping the incision is estimated. This skin is excised in a double triangle pattern so that a lateral lift can be given to the replaced skin (Plate 10-2, *G*). The septum is not sutured. The wound is closed with interrupted 6-0 mild chromic sutures. At times it may be necessary to trim skin in the lateral canthus (Plate 10-2, *H*).

No dressings are applied postoperatively. Application of cold compresses is begun in the recovery room to decrease swelling. Patients are advised to keep their lids out of direct sunlight for several months.

A possible complication of lower lid blepharoplasty is ectropion resulting from lid flaccidity. This should be evaluated preoperatively and a horizontal shortening procedure performed at the time of surgery. Cysts and suture tunnels that develop can be easily treated with excision or light cautery done in the office.

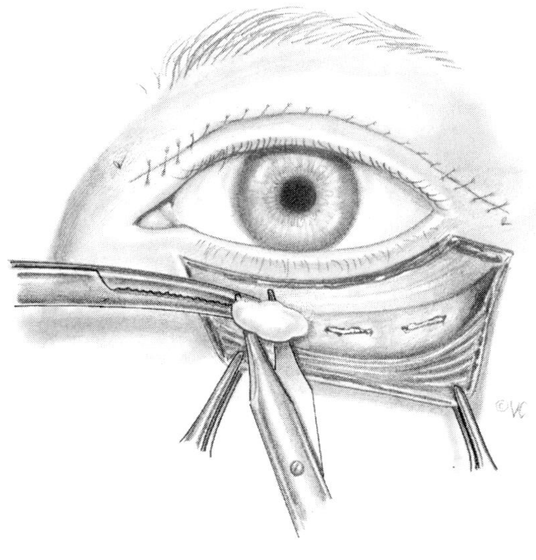

E, Careful clamping of fat.

F, Fat pads cauterized.

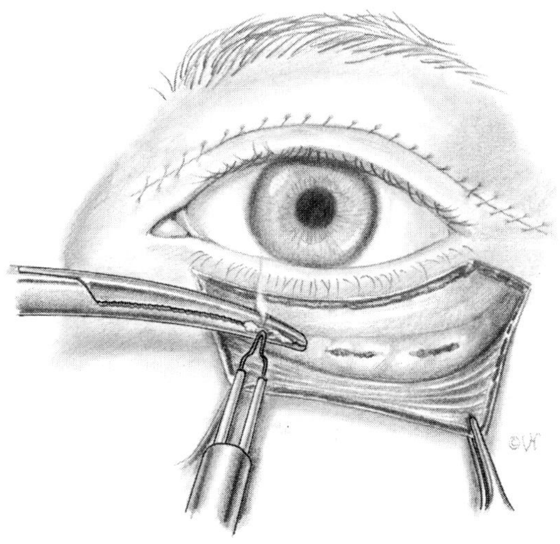

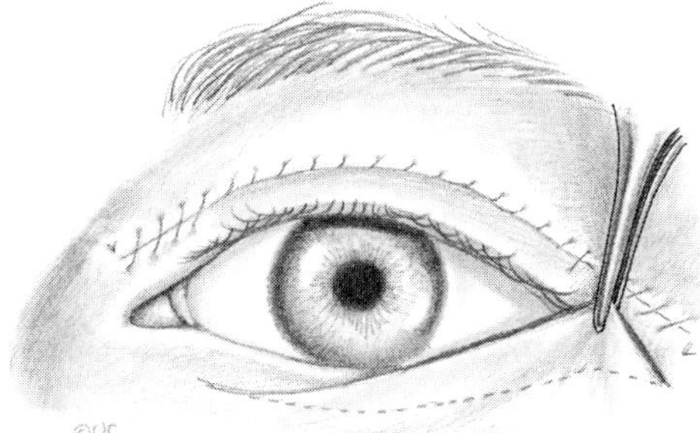

G, Excess skin marked and excised.

H, Lid incision closed with 6-0 absorbable suture.

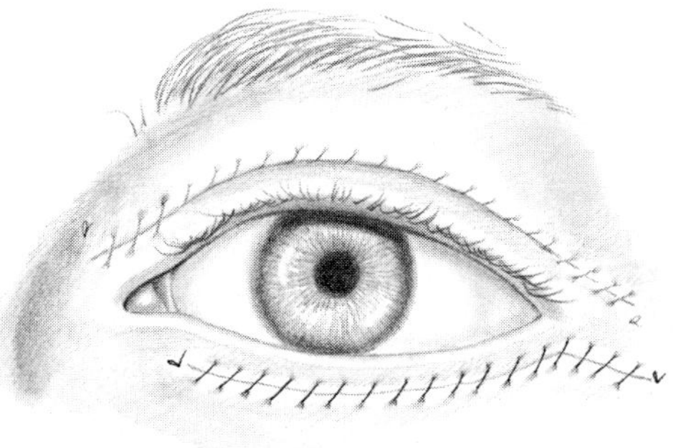

CHAPTER 11

LACRIMAL GLAND SURGERY

The lacrimal gland is located in the lacrimal fossa of the frontal bone, under the superior temporal rim of the orbit. The gland is divided into two lobes, the orbital and palpebral lobes, by the lateral horn of the levator aponeurosis.

Reflex tear secretion is derived from the main lacrimal gland and its palpebral portion. The orbital portion of the gland has four or five ducts that empty above the border of the lateral tarsus. The 15 to 40 ducts of the palpebral portion empty into a common duct, which empties near the main ducts. Excision of the palpebral portion of the gland will most certainly destroy the ducts from the main gland. While the orbital portion of the gland is firmly supported by multiple ligaments in its fossa, the palpebral portion is not and may prolapse downward.

The palpebral lobe of the lacrimal gland can prolapse anteriorly, creating a bulge in the upper eyelid laterally. The orbital lobe is more firmly attached and will usually remain in place. However, blepharochalasis is associated with prolapse of the orbital lobe of the lacrimal gland.

The lacrimal gland is replaced into the lacrimal fossa by fixating it to the periosteum of the orbital rim. An incision is made along the superior lid crease from the middle of the lid laterally to the orbital rim (Plate 11-1, *A*). The upper aspect of the incision is dissected deep to the orbicularis, to the superior orbital rim. The orbital septum is identified and incised (Plate 11-1, *B* and *C*). The incision through the orbital septum is made 2 mm below the orbital rim to allow for its adequate closure.

The lacrimal gland is brought through the incision by applying gentle pressure on the globe (Plate 11-1, *D*). The gland is pinkish gray to yellow, multilobulated, and contained within a tough, diaphanous membrane. It must be differentiated from the yellow, nonlobulated orbital fat. A biopsy of the gland may be performed if there is suspicion of a malignancy.

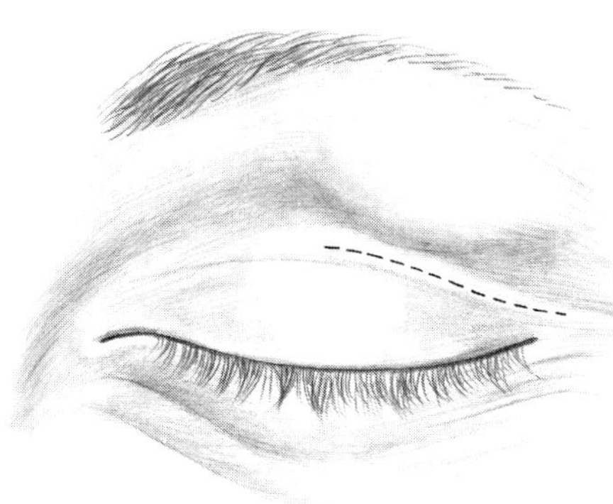

A, Suspension of prolapsed lacrimal gland. Area to be incised is marked at the superior orbital rim.

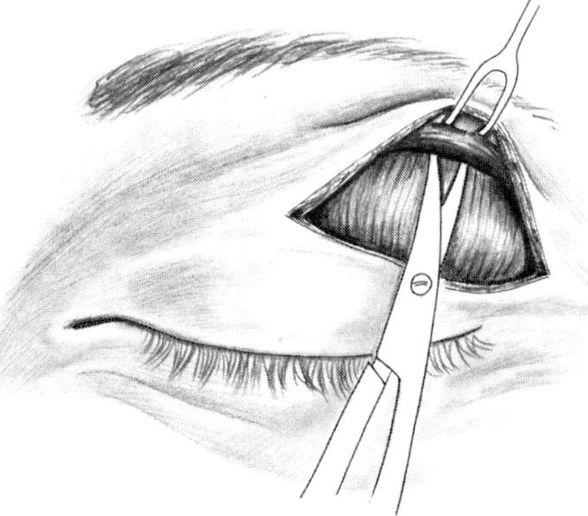

B, The lid is incised, and the dissection is carried down to the orbital septum.

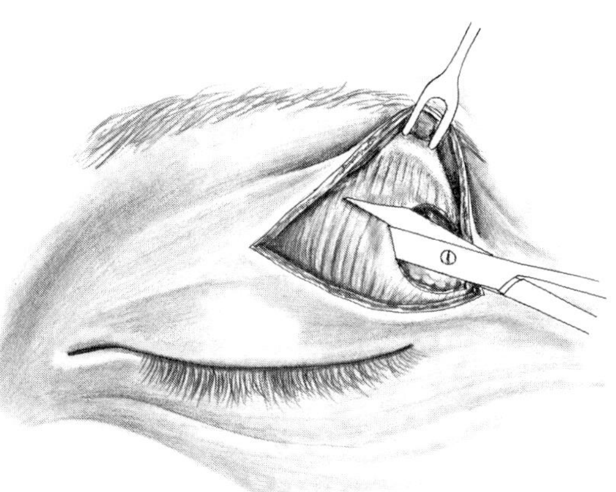

C, The orbital septum is incised.

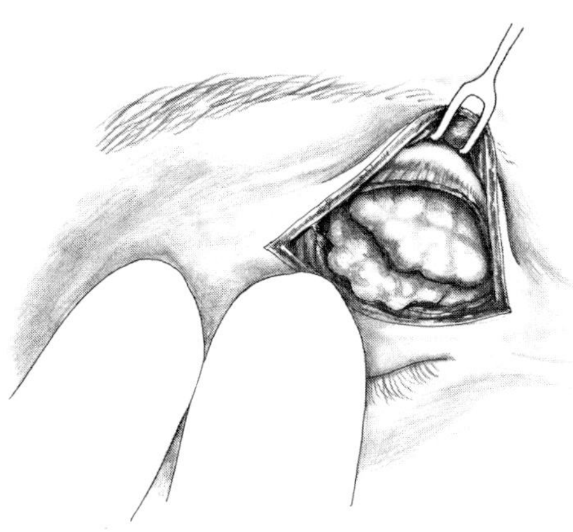

D, The prolapsed lacrimal gland is exposed.

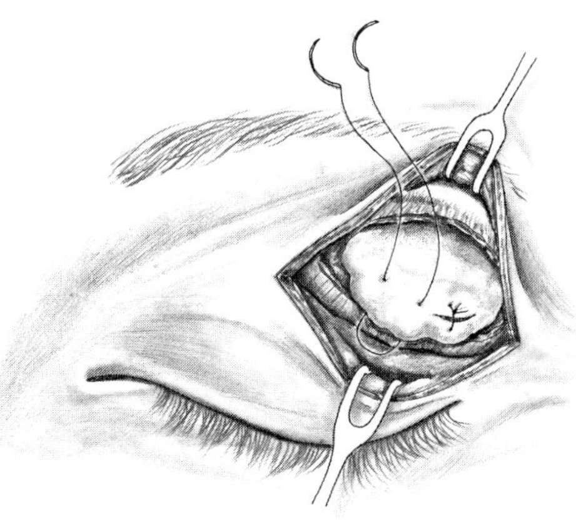

E, A double-armed suture is placed through the gland.

The gland is grasped and both needles of a double-armed 5-0 prolene suture are passed through its anterior portion (Plate 11-1, *E*). The gland is retracted inferiorly, and the two needles are passed posterior to anterior through the periosteum of the roof of the lacrimal fossa to form a mattress suture (Plate 11-1, *F*). The suture is pulled gently to replace the lacrimal gland into position within the lacrimal fossa (Plate 11-1, *G* and *H*). The septum is closed with interrupted 5-0 Vicryl sutures (Plate 11-1, *I*). Excess skin may be draped over the incision and excised as indicated (Plate 11-1, *J*). The skin is closed with interrupted 6-0 mild chromic sutures (Plate 11-1, *K*). To allow observation for any evidence of orbital hemorrhage, the eye is not patched.

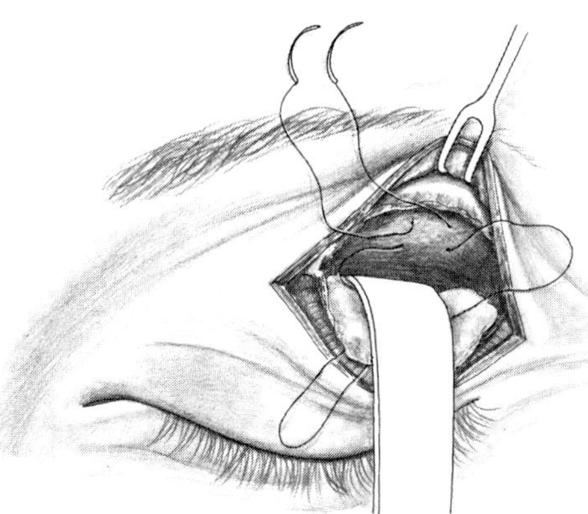

F, The suture is inserted into the roof of the lacrimal fossa.

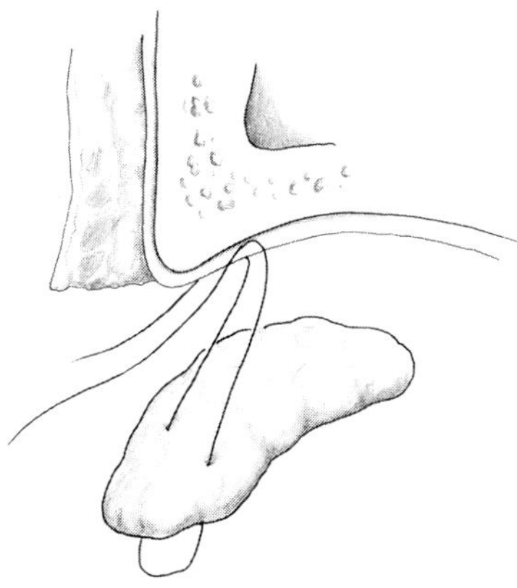

G, Sagittal view of placement of suspension suture.

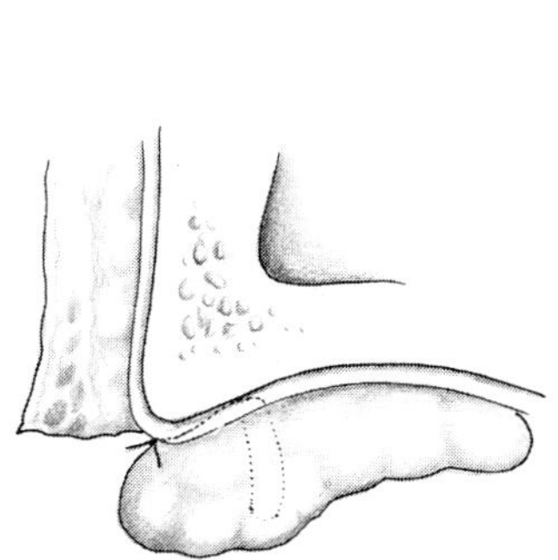

H, Sagittal view of gland suspended in fossa.

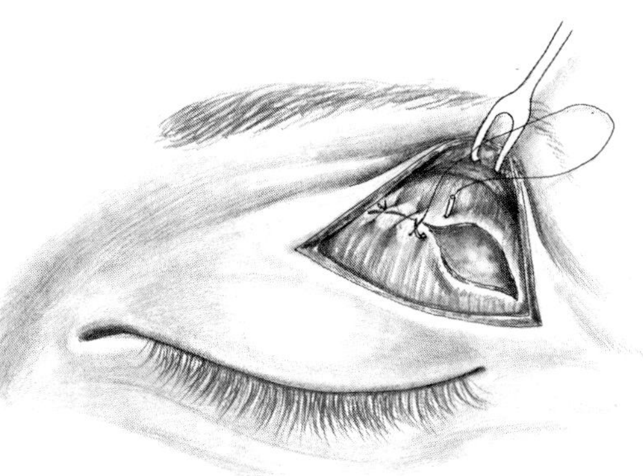

I, Closure of orbital septum.

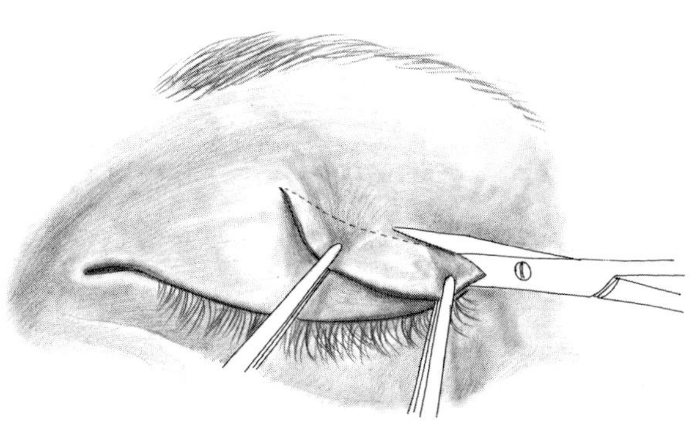

J, Excision of overlapping skin.

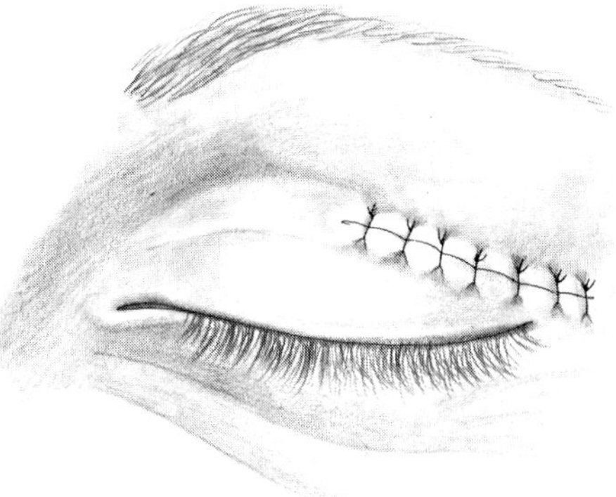

K, Skin closure with interrupted sutures.

CHAPTER 12

DACRYOCYSTORHINOSTOMY OF THE LACRIMAL EXCRETORY SYSTEM

A dacryocystorhinostomy (DCR) is indicated if the lacrimal outflow system proximal to the lacrimal sac is patent and there is an obstruction within the sac or nasolacrimal duct. Prior to performance of a DCR, a nasal examination is needed to evaluate the patient for the possibility of nasal pathology that will cause the fistula created by the surgery to close. Dacryoscintography can be helpful to evaluate for the presence of a dacryolith or neoplastic obstruction.

Local anesthesia with a 50:50 mixture of 2% lidocaine and 0.75% Marcaine, both with 1:100,000 epinephrine, is preferred for this procedure. The entire medial canthal area, including periosteum in the lacrimal fossa, is infiltrated. All four walls of the ipsilateral nasal passage are packed with gauze soaked in 4% cocaine, preferably under direct visualization. They may also be injected with the local anesthetic. If general anesthesia is required, the area of dissection should be infiltrated in an identical manner, with the same solution. The nasal passage should also be packed as described.

The incision is made over the medial inferior orbital rim (Plate 12-1, *A*). It extends from just below the medial canthal tendon laterally approximately 15 mm. It may be lengthened further as required during the procedure. The globe is protected by wedging the nondominant index finger under the anterior lacrimal crest during the incision, which is carried down to the periosteum in a single pass. Meticulous hemostasis is maintained with bipolar cautery and thermal cautery as indicated.

The incision is retracted, and the periosteum just anterior to the anterior lacrimal crest is incised with a scalpel. The periosteum is retracted posteriorly over the anterior lacrimal crest to the posterior lacrimal crest (Plate 12-1, *B*). The periosteal elevator is then used to reflect the sac temporally, away from the lacrimal groove. A ⅛-inch cottonoid soaked in 4% cocaine is placed between the lacrimal sac and the lacrimal fossa and allowed to sit for a few minutes.

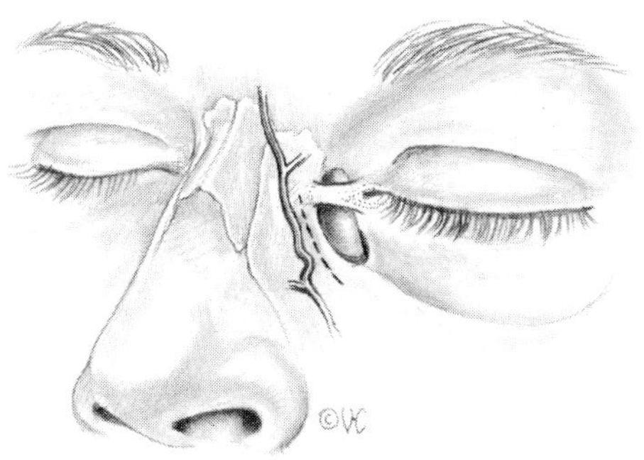

A, Area to be incised is outlined on the underlying bony landmarks.

B, Periosteum incised and lacrimal sac reflected posteriorly.

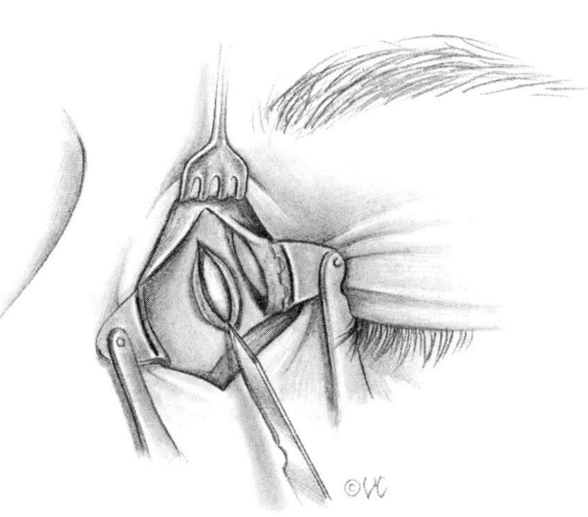

The cottonoid is removed, and the posterior superior lacrimal fossa is penetrated to the anterior ethmoids with a drill or hemostat (Plate 12-1, *C*). The opening is enlarged anteriorly and inferiorly with progressively larger neurosurgical rongeurs until it is slightly larger than the size of a dime (Plate 12-1, *D* to *G*). Care is taken to preserve the nasal mucosa during this step. The primary cause of failure of this procedure is thought to be closure of an inadequate bony ostomy. The rongeurs should be used to cut the bone out by the direct cutting action of their jaws. They should not be used to grasp the bone and pry it out. Prying out bone in this area can cause severe bleeding and tears in the lamina cribrosa.

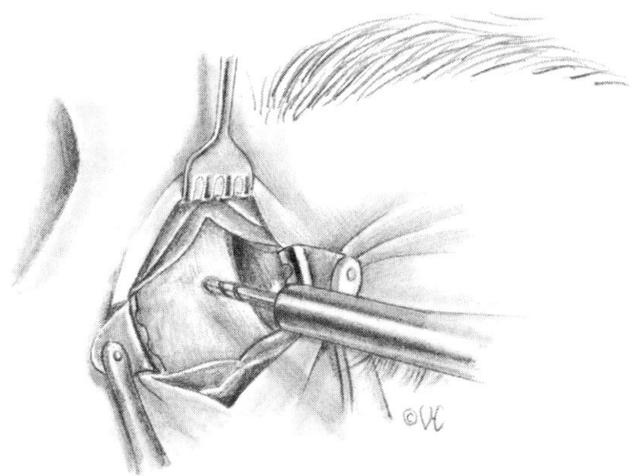

C, Bone is penetrated with drill or small hemostat.

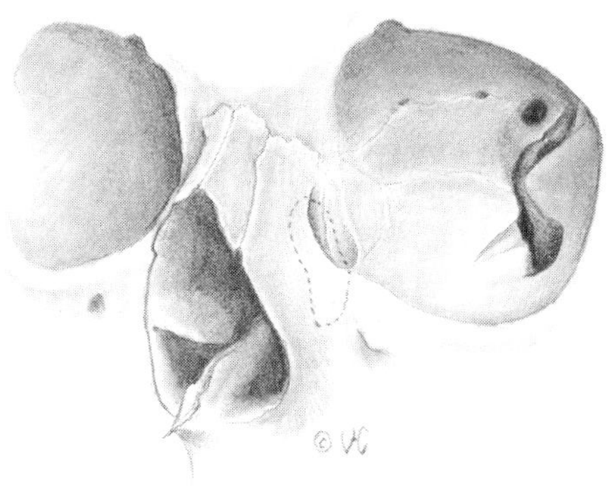

D, Area of osteotomy to be created.

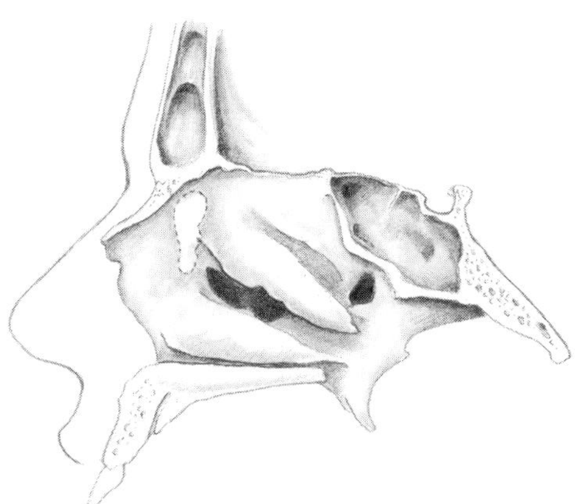

E, Osteotomy made into anterior middle turbinate

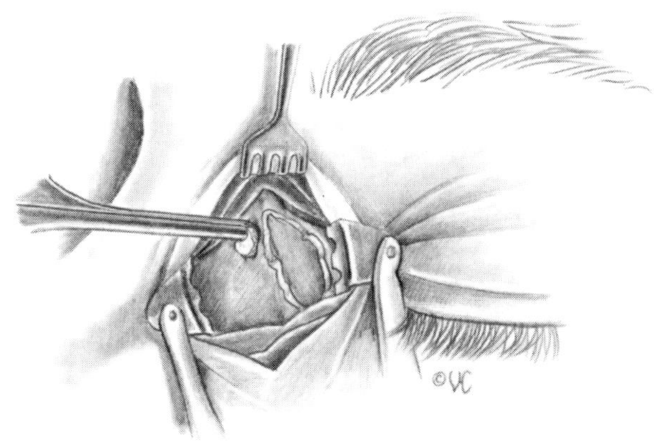

F, Rongeurs used to enlarge osteotomy.

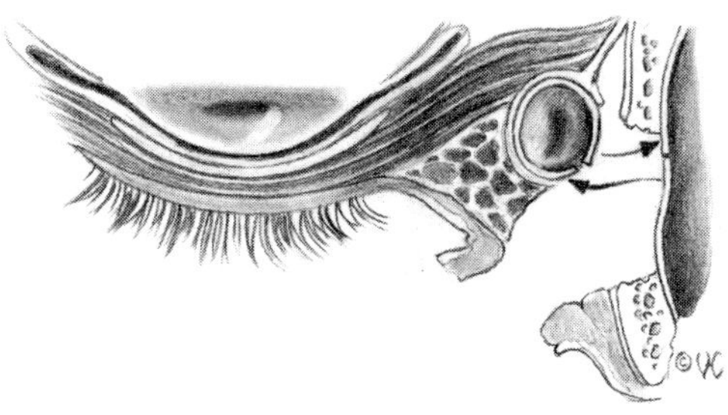

G, Horizontal section demonstrating osteotomy medial to lacrimal sac.

A no. 12 Bard-Parker blade is used to incise the nasal mucosa and create a U-shaped flap to form an anterior mucosal flap (Plate 12-1, *H*). The upper and lower puncta are dilated, and a lacrimal probe is passed into the lacrimal sac. The same blade is used to create an anterior U-shaped lacrimal sac flap, a mirror image of the nasal mucosal flap. The nasal packing is removed. The upper and lower canaliculi are intubated with Silastic tubing, which is brought out the nose and tied together (Plate 12-1, *I* and *J*). A single square knot is tied in the tubing, and the tubing is cut ⅛-inch long and allowed to retract into the nose.

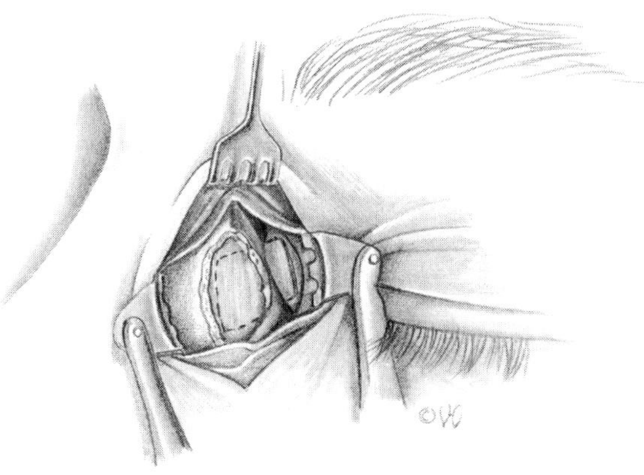

H, U-shaped mucosal flap is outlined.

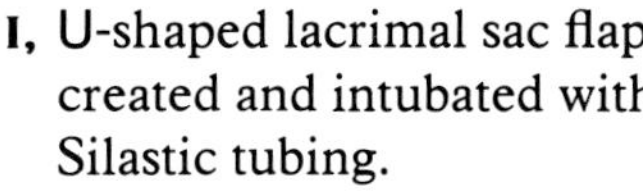

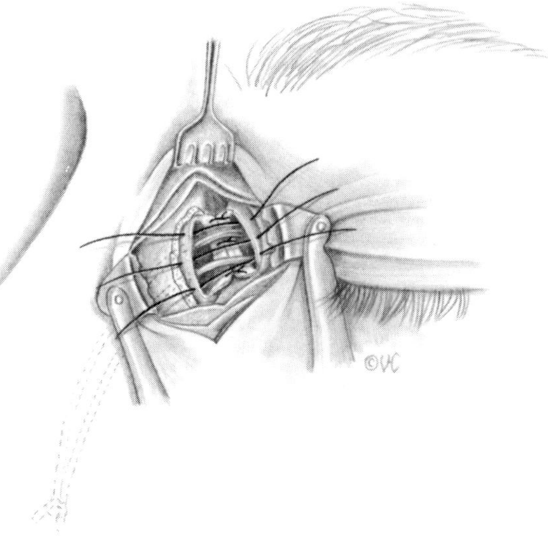

I, U-shaped lacrimal sac flap created and intubated with Silastic tubing.

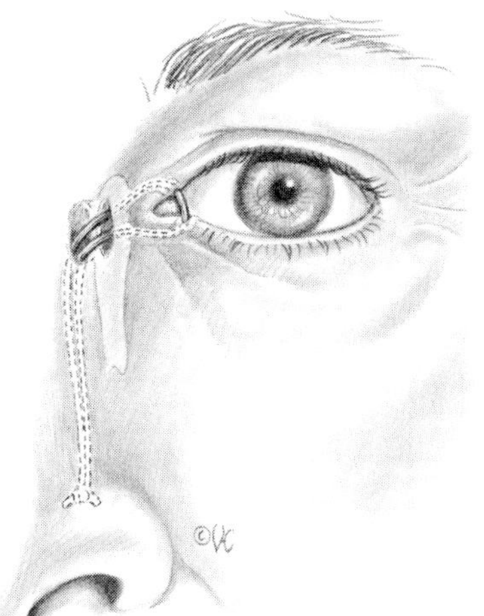

J, Crawford tubing tied in nose.

The mucosal flaps are sutured together with a multiple 5-0 Vicryl horizontal sutures (Plate 12-1, *K*). The muscular layer is closed with 5-0 Vicryl sutures (Plate 12-1, *L*). The skin is closed with interrupted 6-0 mild chromic sutures (Plate 12-1, *M*). The eye is pressure patched with antibiotic ointment.

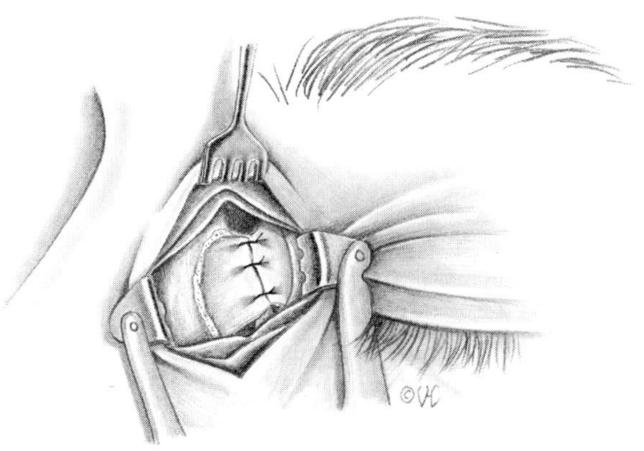

K, Nasal mucosal flap sutured to lacrimal sac flap.

L, Muscle layer closed with 5-0 Vicryl suture.

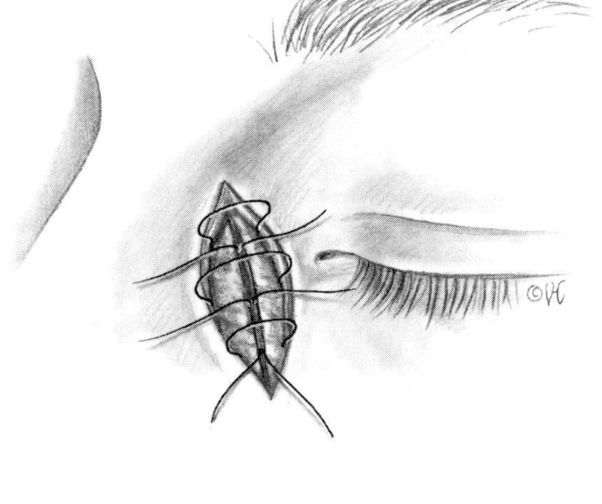

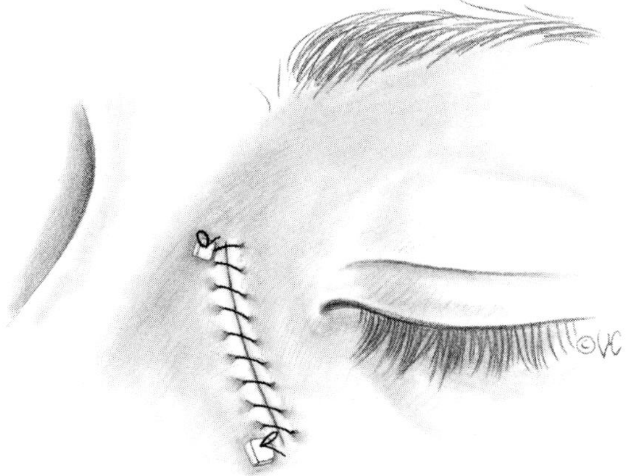

M, Skin closed with interrupted 6-0 mild chromic sutures.

CHAPTER 13

BLEPHAROPTOSIS

The preoperative evaluation of the ptosis patient is probably as significant to the treatment of this condition as the type of surgery and the skill with which it is performed. One must begin by differentiating between acquired and congenital ptosis. An accurate history must be obtained. The amount of ptosis surgery required for congenital ptosis is greater than that required for acquired ptosis. Performing an unsuitable procedure will lead to an unsatisfactory result.

A complete ophthalmologic examination must be performed. It must include a careful study of muscle balance to rule out the possibility of a hypotropia causing a pseudoptosis. A Schirmer test for adequacy of lacrimal production should be performed in case an overcorrection results, even transiently. An estimate should be made of levator function by measuring the interpalpebral fissure in primary position, and in up and down gaze. During these measurements, the action of the frontalis muscle should be inhibited by exerting external pressure on the brow. Patients with good levator function, greater than 12 mm, generally require less correction than patients with less than 5 mm of levator function. In congenital ptosis with less than 3 mm of levator function, a frontalis suspension usually produces the best results.

The patient should be tested for an adequate Bell's phenomenon. Good elevation of the globe during forced closure of the lids is a good sign that any postoperative lagophthalmos will be well tolerated. The patient should be examined for congenital or traumatic fibrosis in the upper lid. A lagophthalmos on down-gaze with a mechanical obstruction to active extension of the lid will mean further lagophthalmos if ptosis surgery is performed. Photo documentation of the patient's eyes and lids is an essential portion of the preoperative evaluation.

A patient may have an apparent ptosis in one eye as compared with the other when the apparently normal eye is actually proptosed. The possibility of this should be kept in mind and properly evaluated. The presence of a Marcus Gunn phenomenon, or a jaw-winking phenomenon, should be ascertained by history and observation. Failure to note this relatively common condition in ptosis patients could have disastrous consequences.

The neurologic status of the patient should be checked if necessary. Edrophonium (Tensilon) testing for ocular myasthenia may be indicated. Neurogenic ptosis resulting from third-nerve injury usually requires frontalis suspension.

Finally, it should be explained to the patient or parent that ptosis surgery is more an art than a science and that, even in the best of hands, complications can and do result.

Of the many ptosis procedures available in the literature, the four we find most practical in handling almost all cases of ptosis are (1) the frontalis fixation, (2) the external levator resection, (3) the levator advancement, and (4) the Fasanella-Servat procedure.

In cases of external ophthalmoplegia, congenital ptosis with minimal levator function, aberrant nerve regeneration, or mechanical restriction of the lid, the suspension of the lid margin from the frontalis muscle is a reliable method of ptosis correction. Even in cases with poor or absent Bell's phenomenon resulting from extraocular muscle restriction or paresis, this procedure is usually well tolerated, and offers the advantage of simple removal of the supporting sutures if desired. We have performed a large number of these procedures using 4-0 Supramid suture swaged onto a ski needle, and only rarely have we had to remove the suture in cases of wound infection or granuloma. Autogenous or banked fascia lata is also an excellent material for use in this procedure. The configuration we prefer for this procedure is the double rhomboid.

With the patient under general anesthesia, three stab incisions are made with a razor knife above the brow, in the central, medial, and lateral areas. Then, with adequate protection for the globe, preferably a bone plate, three incisions are made about 2 mm above the lash line, down to the tarsus.

The ski needle with the swaged-on 4-0 Supramid is then inserted through the temporal brow incision and moved downward to be withdrawn from the lateral lid incision (Plate 13-1, *A*). The needle is reinserted, moved medially, and withdrawn from the central incision. It is then passed superiorly and withdrawn from the central brow incision. Finally, it is reinserted into the central brow incision and withdrawn from the original temporal brow incision. A similar rhomboid is created on the medial aspect of the lid, the central incisions being utilized a second time.

The sutures are then tied in the superior temporal and superior nasal brow sites. By adjusting the tension of the suture, the surgeon can set the height of the lid. The knots are inserted into the depth of the wound, and the lid assumes its new position (Plate 13-1, *B*). The superior superficial incisions are closed with interrupted 6-0 mild chromic sutures. The procedure can be repeated on the contralateral upper lid.

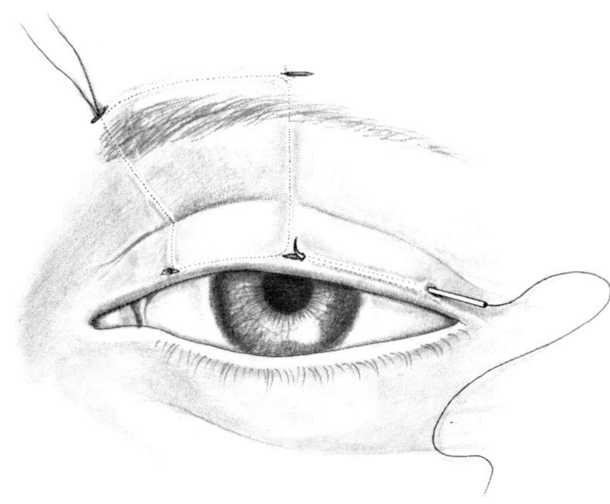

A, Ski needle used to carry Supramid suture through stab incisions.

B, Completion of double rhomboid–type fixation.

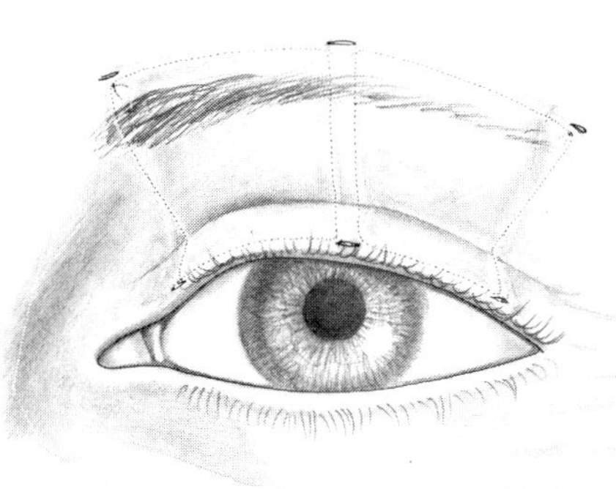

Banked fascia lata is now commercially available. Its insertion is slightly different and is described below.

The eyelid and brow are injected with 1% lidocaine with 1:100,000 epinephrine to aid in hemostasis during general anesthesia. Three stab incisions are made with a knife blade above the brow, in the central, medial, and lateral areas. Then, with adequate protection for the globe, two eyelid incisions are made through the skin and pretarsal orbicularis muscles. Scissor dissection then carefully exposes the tarsal plate (Plate 13-2, *A*).

If both eyelids are being operated on, the second brow and eyelid incisions should be made at this time. An assistant may then maintain pressure on the opposite incisions while the surgeon works. Placement of hemostatic collagen material aids significantly in hemostasis.

A Jaeger lid plate is placed under the eyelid and brought into contact with the orbital rim to ensure protection of the globe. A Wright fascia needle is then passed through the temporal incision, passed just anterior to septum in the lid tissues, and brought out through the temporal eyelid incision. Fascia lata is then loaded into the eye of the Wright needle and the fascia is brought out from temporal brow incision (Plate 13-2, *B*). A 2-cm segment is pulled out of the temporal incision. The Wright needle is then passed through the two lid incisions just anterior to the tarsal plate, which allows passage of the fascia lata underneath the pretarsal orbicularis (Plate 13-2, *C*).

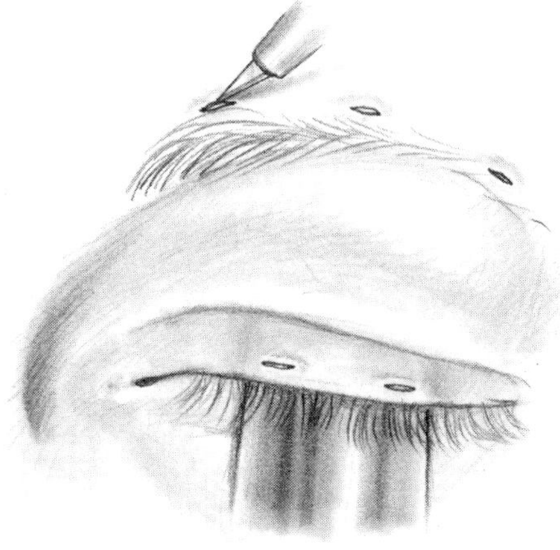

A, Brow and eyelid stab incisions are made.

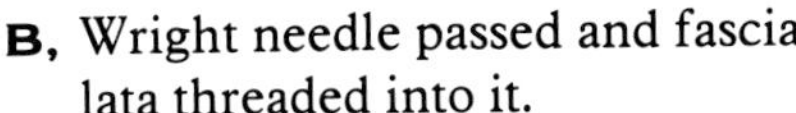

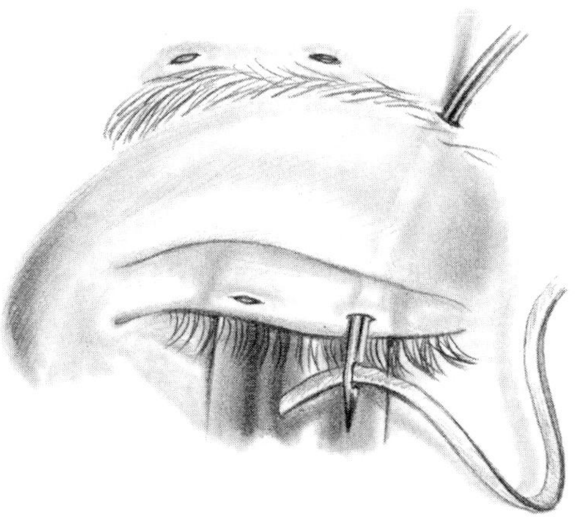

B, Wright needle passed and fascia lata threaded into it.

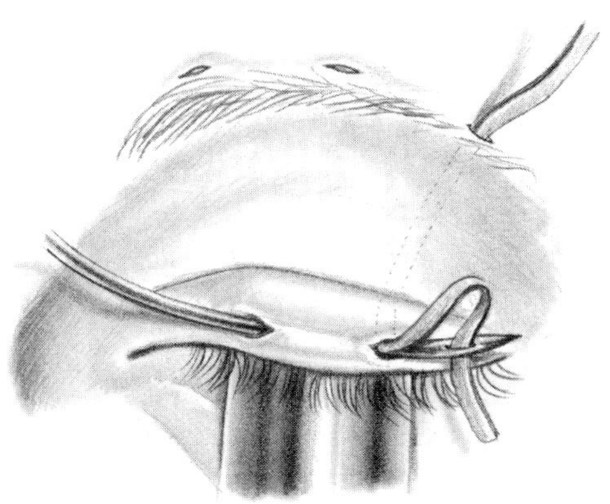

C, Fascia lata threaded through lid.

The Wright needle is then passed from the nasal brow incision to the nasal lid incision, and the fascia lata is brought out of the nasal brow incision (Plate 13-2, *D*). The Wright needle is passed from the central brow incision to both central and nasal brow incisions, which will allow the fascia lata to be brought out of the central brow incision (Plate 13-2, *E* and *F*).

The eyelid is elevated just to the point of overcorrection. The fascia lata is then secured with 5-0 prolene. The suture is interwoven with knots in the fascia lata to prevent slippage (Plate 13-2, *G*). The fascia lata knot is then placed deep in the central brow incision, allowing the lid to drop into contact with the globe. The brow and eyelid incisions are closed with one or two 6-0 mild chromic sutures.

After use of either Supramid or banked fascia lata, a light dressing is applied and then removed after 24 hours. Artificial tears are used frequently postoperatively, with a bland ointment instilled at night. The patient generally tolerates the procedure well.

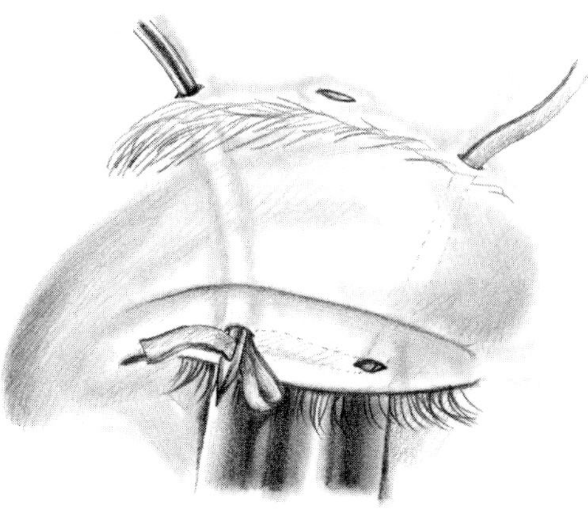

D, Fascia lata brought through brow incision.

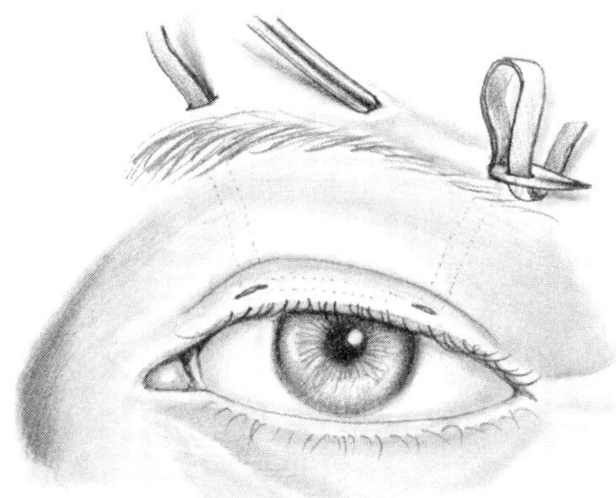

E, Fascia lata passed from temporal to central brow incisions.

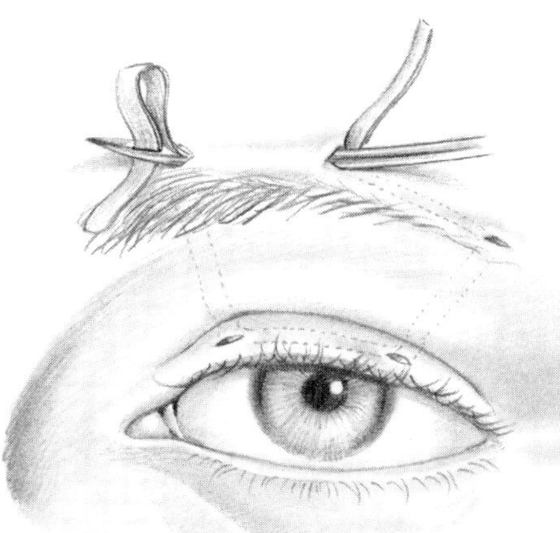

F, Fascia lata passed from nasal brow incision to central brow incision.

G, Lid elevated and fascia lata secured.

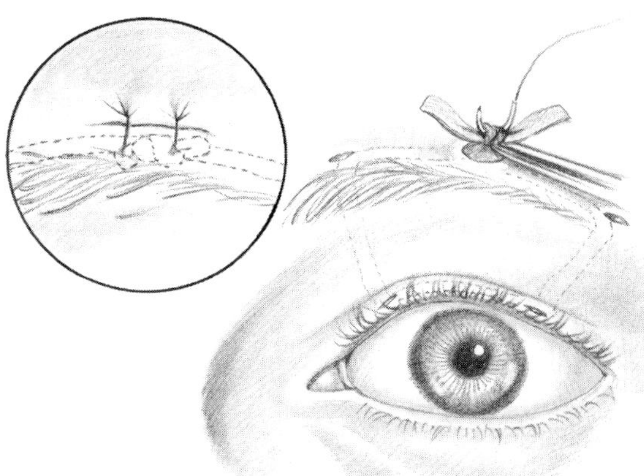

The anterior approach to resection or advancement of the levator aponeurosis is an excellent procedure in cases of congenital ptosis. The exposure of the aponeurosis in congenital ptosis is unsurpassed by any other procedure and permits resection and tarsal advancement enough to correct almost any amount of ptosis. It allows the lid to be set at any desired level with easy and directly visible accessibility to all of the lid structures.

General anesthesia is used for very young children. However, the local injection of 2% lidocaine with 1:100,000 epinephrine permits the correction to be gauged in the operating room. Through experience we have found that it is best to seek a slight over-correction; otherwise, the lid level will tend to fall too low.

A cotton-tipped applicator is used to elevate the lid margin and estimate the level of the supratarsal crease, which is often absent in cases of ptosis.

The supratarsal crease is then designated with a marking pencil. The area is infil-trated with a local anesthetic regardless of the type of anesthetic used, because it pro-vides hydraulic dissection of the skin from the orbicularis and aids in hemostasis, as well as producing akinesia.

With the lid stretched, a razor knife is used to incise the designated area, which is dissected inferiorly between the skin and orbicularis to just above the lash line (Plate 13-3, *A*).

Skin hooks or forceps are then used to grasp the lower skin flap, and with the lid on stretch, the superior one third of the pretarsal orbicularis is excised.

With the lid extended downward, scissors are used to perforate the orbital septum (Plate 13-3, *B* and *C*). If the incision has been made in the correct plane, the white sheath of the aponeurosis is visible with preaponeurotic fat lying above it. Dissection is carried horizontally in both directions.

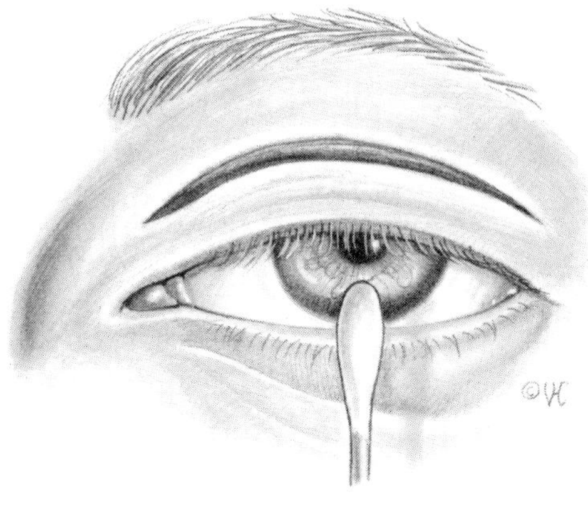

A, Cotton-tipped applicator used to gauge level of supratarsal crease and site to be incised.

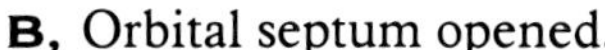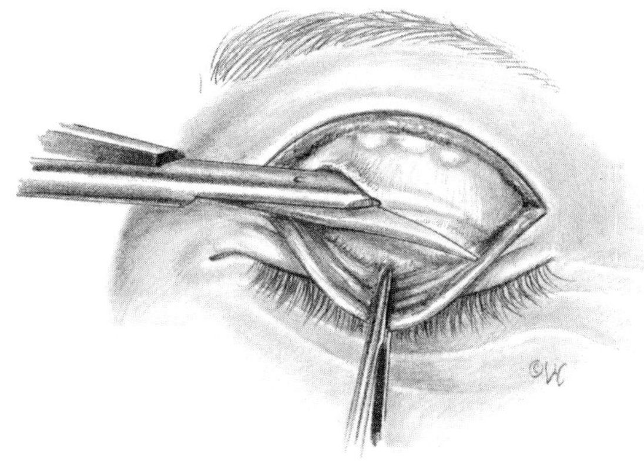

B, Orbital septum opened.

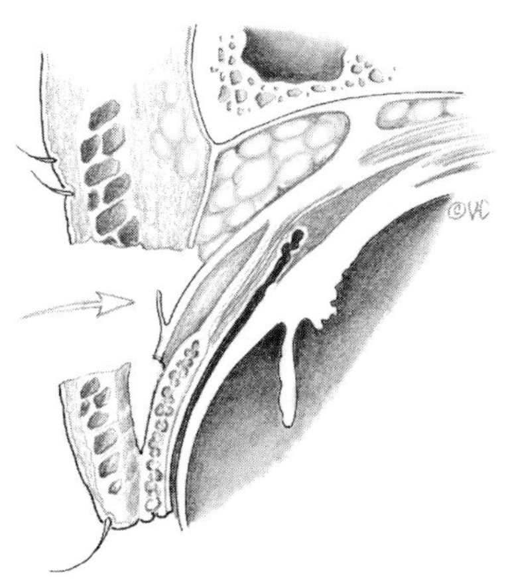

C, Sagittal view of orbital septum opened; tarsus exposed.

Conjunctiva is then ballooned away from Müller's fibers. It is carefully dissected free from the muscle layer (Plate 13-3, *D*).

A double-armed 5-0 Novafil suture is then placed in the midtarsus to a depth of about one-half the tarsal plate (Plate 13-3, *E*). The suture is placed with a 5-mm bite horizontally across tarsus (Plate 13-3, *F*) and brought through the levator and Müller's muscle in mattress fashion (Plate 13-3, *G*).

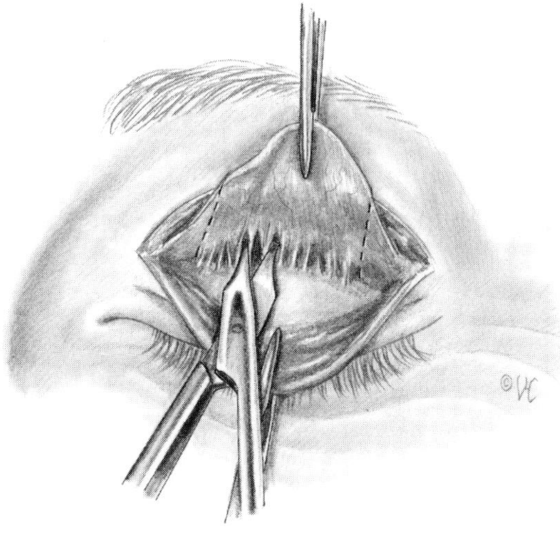

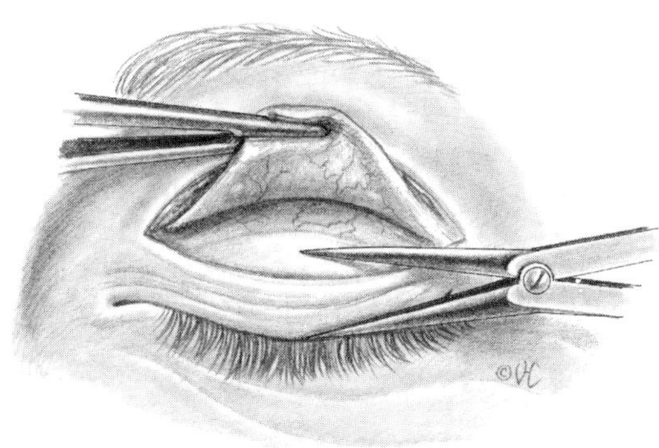

D, Levator grasped and Müller's muscle dissected free from conjunctiva.

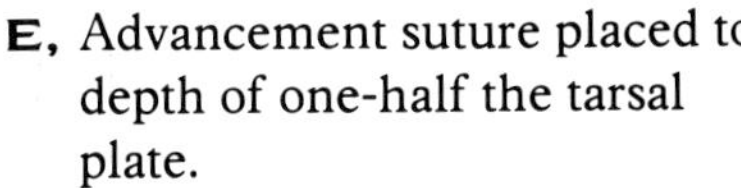

E, Advancement suture placed to depth of one-half the tarsal plate.

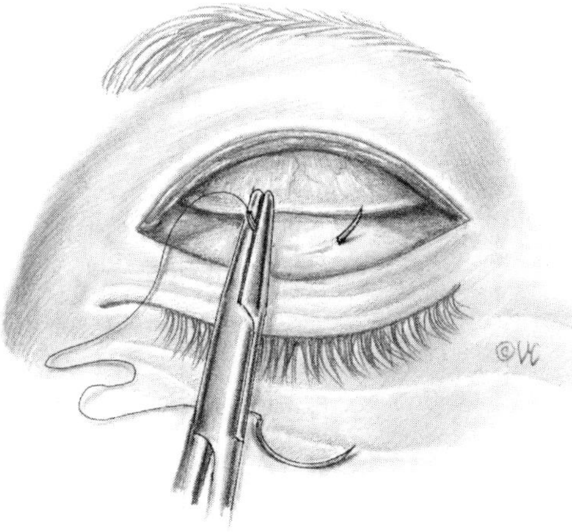

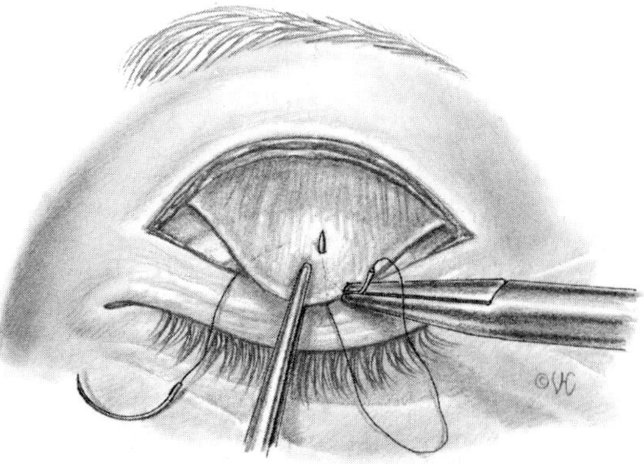

F, Suture is placed with a 5-mm horizontal bite.

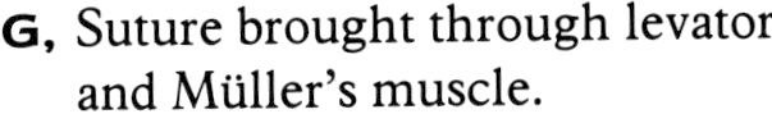

G, Suture brought through levator and Müller's muscle.

The suture is tightened but not tied, and the lid level is evaluated. This lid margin should be slightly above the desired level. If the lid is not at the desired level, the suture is removed and reinserted until the proper level is reached (Plate 13-3, *H*). Further lateral and medial sutures can be placed if desired. The excess levator is measured and excised.

For skin closure 6-0 chromic sutures are placed full thickness through the inferior skin edge to grasp the levator aponeurosis and exit through the superior skin edge. This creates an excellent lid fold and does not require suture removal in children (Plate 13-3, *I* and *J*).

Postoperatively, especially in congenital ptosis, patients should be observed for corneal irritation caused by lagophthalmos and treated accordingly with artificial tears and bland ointments.

In the event of undercorrection, the procedure should be repeated. If the levator function was poor to begin with, a frontalis fixation eventually may be necessary.

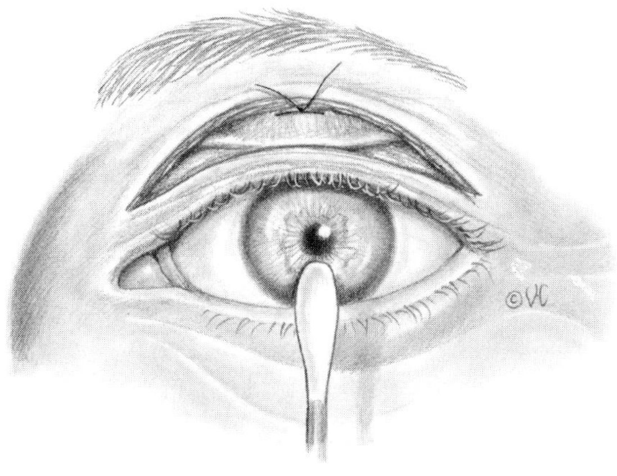

H, Suture tied and lid level evaluated.

I, Wound closed with interrupted sutures.

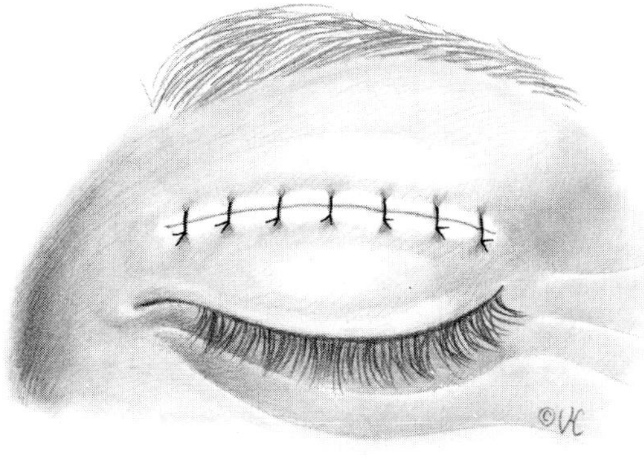

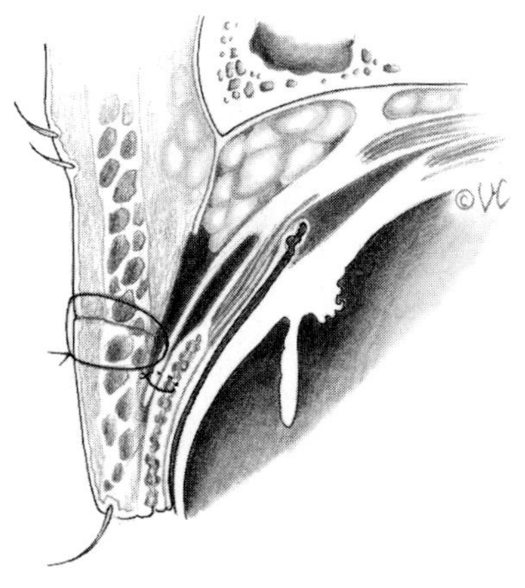

J, Sagittal view of wound closure.

Blepharoptosis is a common sequela of aging and trauma. It is especially common after intraocular surgery in people over 60 years of age. In someone with a levator function of 6 mm or greater, the blepharoptosis is corrected most effectively by an external approach. We strongly favor the technique described below. It allows the lid to be set at the optimum height intraoperatively, regardless of the cause of the ptosis.

The procedure is best accomplished with local anesthesia and short-acting intravenous sedation. However, after several hundred cases with local anesthesia, we have been able to set the lid height with excellent results during general anesthesia. The local anesthetic solution is a 50:50 mixture of 2% lidocaine and 0.75% Marcaine, both with 1:100,000 epinephrine. The injection must be made just below the skin and above the septum to prevent any effect on the levator and Müller's muscles (Plate 13-4, *A*).

Prior to the injection, the incision is marked out in the same manner as with blepharoplasty. The lid is stretched and held in position. The incision is made with a razor knife into the orbicularis, not through it. Curved iris scissors are used to excise the skin and muscle within the incision. Hemostasis is achieved with thermal cautery.

The inferior incision edge is grasped with Castroviejo forceps, and pretarsal skin is dissected off of underlying pretarsal orbicularis with curved iris scissors (Plate 13-4, *B*). While an assistant holds the dissected skin, the pretarsal orbicularis is then excised from the superior third of the tarsus in a horizontal ellipse (Plate 13-4, *C*). Hemostasis is achieved with thermal cautery. Two thermal cautery spots, Tresley spots, are placed partial thickness in the exposed tarsal plate, centered on the pupil, 5 mm apart.

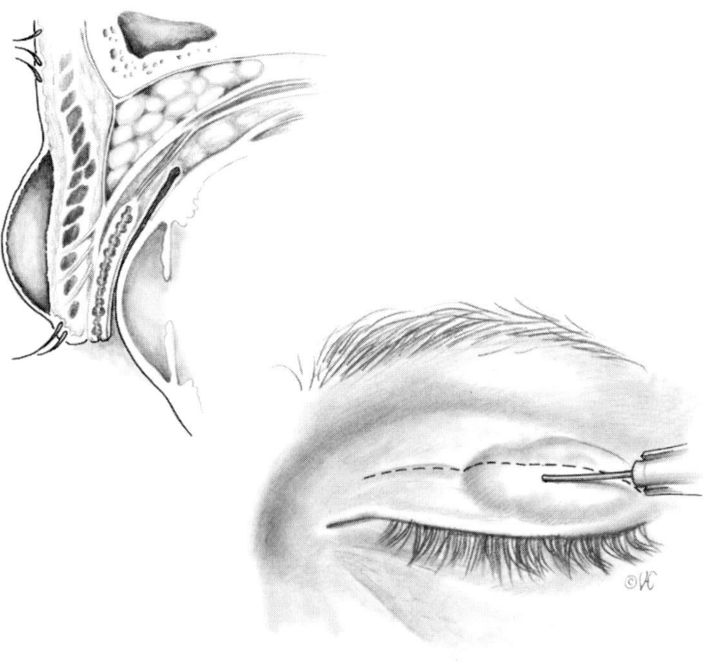

A, Incision site outlined and lid infiltrated with anesthetic solution.

B, Skin dissected from pretarsal orbicularis.

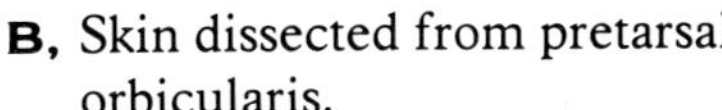

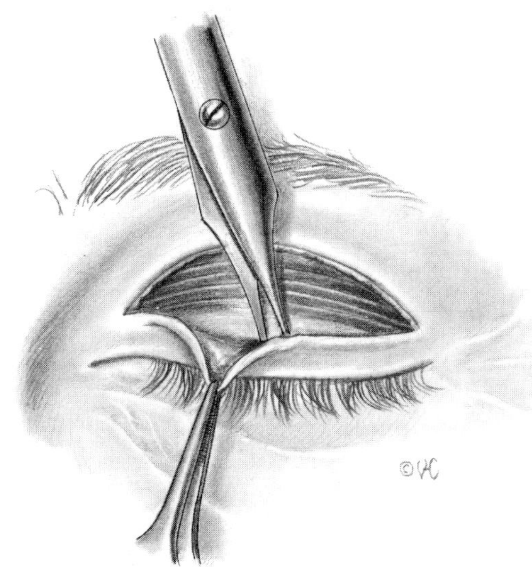

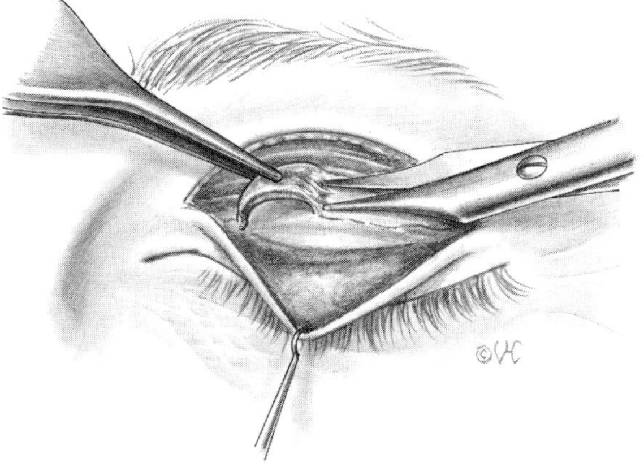

C, Superior third of pretarsal orbicularis is removed tarsus.

The inferior edge of the levator aponeurosis is grasped and gently pulled downward. The septum just below the superior skin incision is grasped and tented upward. The septum is entered with scissors angled downward at a 45-degree angle from the frontal plane (Plate 13-4, *D*). The septum is dissected off the levator aponeurosis sufficiently to expose the levator. The preaponeurotic fat defines the space between the levator and the septum and is used to avoid injuring the levator (Plate 13-4, *E*).

A double-armed, 5-0 Novafil suture is passed between the cautery spots in the tarsus. The lid is everted to confirm only partial-thickness penetration of the tarsus, the Siddens flip. The amount of elevation required is estimated, and both needles are passed through the levator aponeurosis an appropriate distance from the inferior levator edge to elevate the lid margin. The needles are passed through the levator from the undersurface and tied anterior to it with a single throw. The suture knot forms a rhomboid (Plate 13-4, *F*).

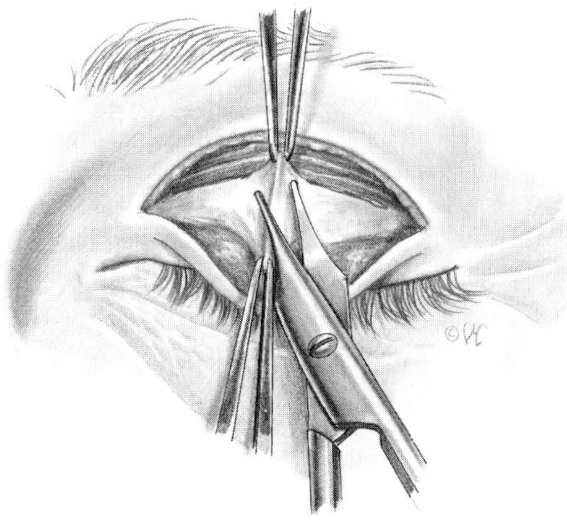

D, Orbital septum is tented upward and incised.

E, Levator exposed, with preaponeurotic fat anterior to it.

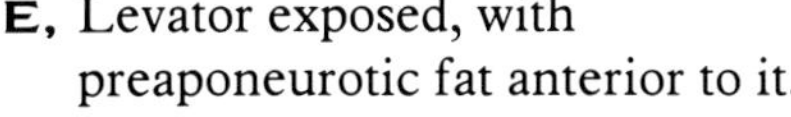

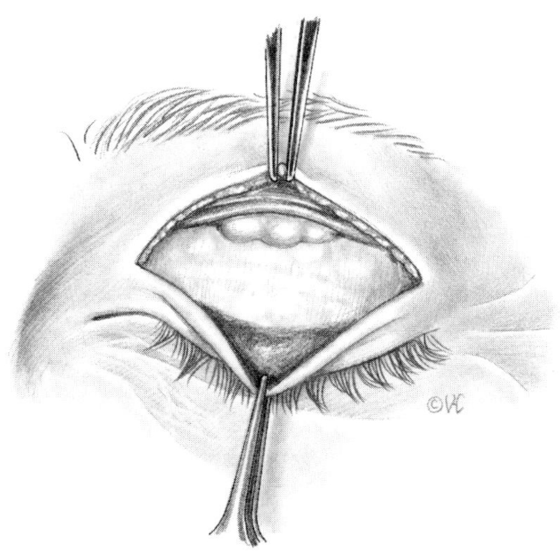

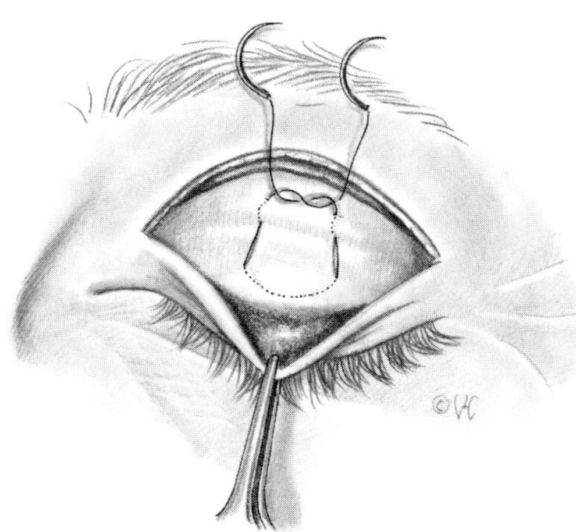

F, Broad-based mattress suture of 5-0 Novafil placed.

The lid height, position, and contour are checked. The single broad-based suture allows simple, effective intraoperative adjustments to the lid (Plate 13-4, *G*). If the lid is too high, the suture is removed from the levator and repassed at a lower point. If the lid is too low, the suture is removed and repassed at a higher point. If the lid is peaked or flat, the intratarsal portion is too narrow or too wide, respectively. After all adjustments are made, the knot is completed with four throws and the suture is cut at the knot. On occasion additional sutures are required temporally and/or medially to establish the optimum lid contour.

The skin is closed and the lid crease re-formed with interrupted 6-0 mild chromic sutures (Plate 13-4, *H*). The crease is re-formed by three cardinal sutures, which are placed laterally, centrally, and medially. Each is passed through the skin along the inferior incision, then through the levator along the superior incision, and finally through the skin along the superior incision. The remainder of the incision is closed with skin-to-skin suture passes. The eye is pressure patched with antibiotic ointment until the following day.

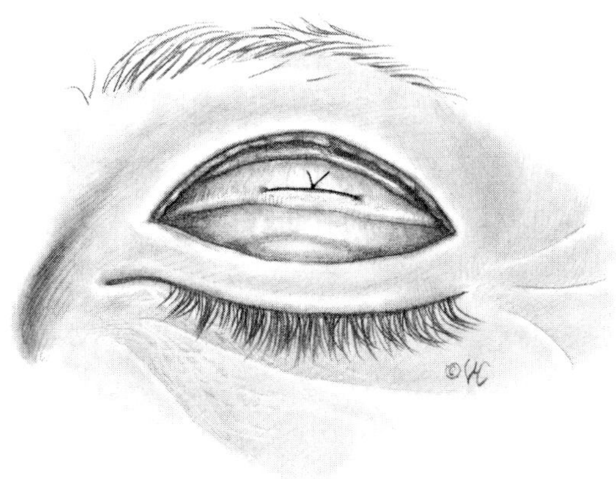

G, Suture tied through levator.

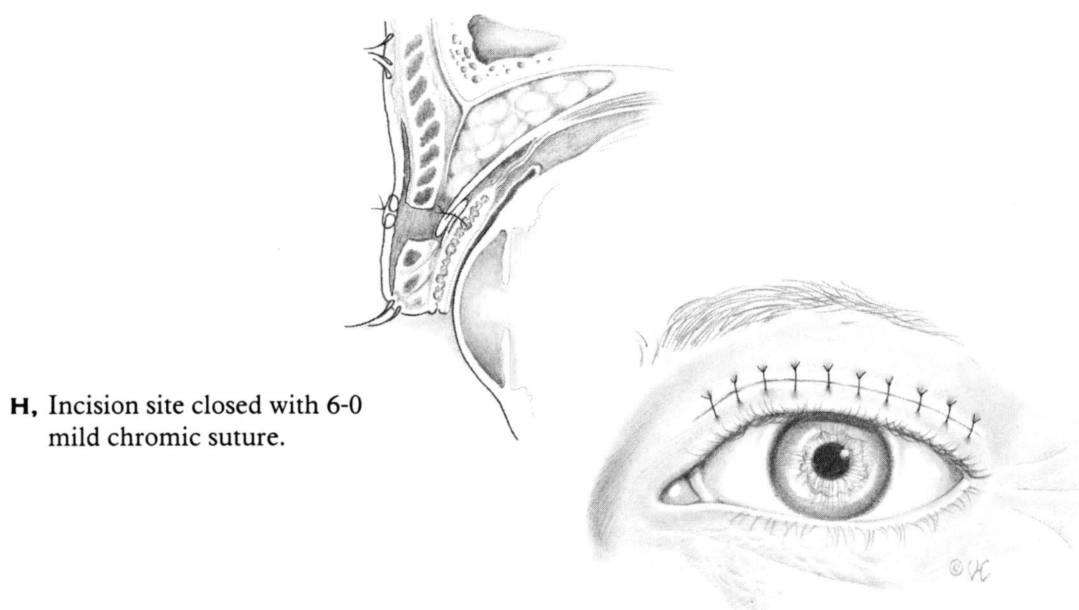

H, Incision site closed with 6-0
mild chromic suture.

In cases of minimal ptosis and good levator function, the Fasanella-Servat procedure is useful. The upper lid is everted and two curved hemostats are placed, one medially and one temporally. Within the hemostats are contained the conjunctiva, the upper-lid retractors, and the superior edge of the tarsus. A 6-0 double-armed monofilament suture is passed full thickness from the external surface of the lid to just under the temporal hemostat (Plate 13-5, *A* and *B*).

The suture is threaded back and forth behind the clamps at a 45-degree angle, with the exit site used as the entrance for the next needle pass (Plate 13-5, *C* and *D*). At the medial end of the everted lid, the suture exits through full thickness to the external surface of the lid (Plate 13-5, *E*).

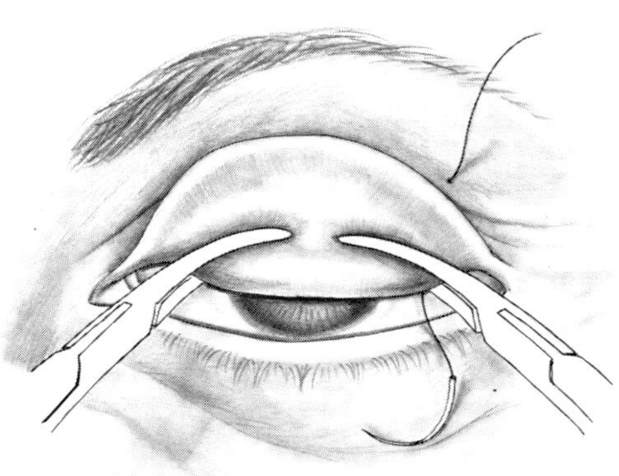

A, Lid everted and curved hemostats placed.

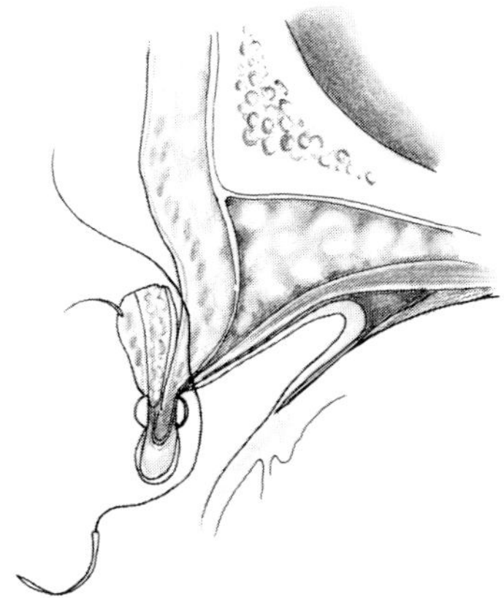

B, Sagittal view of initial suture placement before weaving technique.

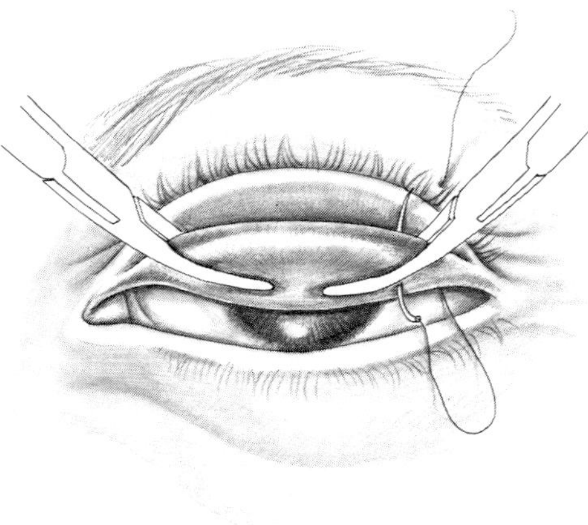

C, Monofilament suture passed full thickness through supratarsal crease to below clamp.

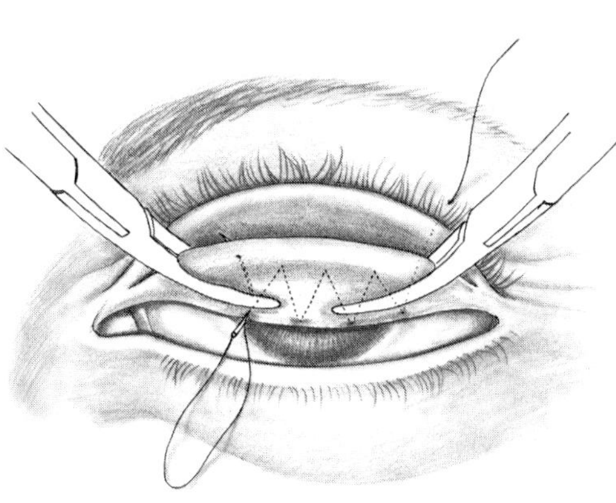

D, Suture woven in back of clamp.

E, Suture through full thickness of lid.

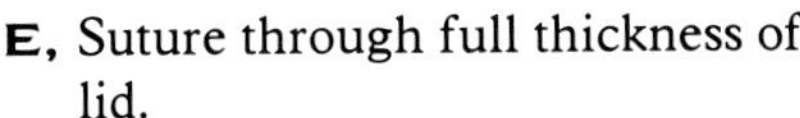

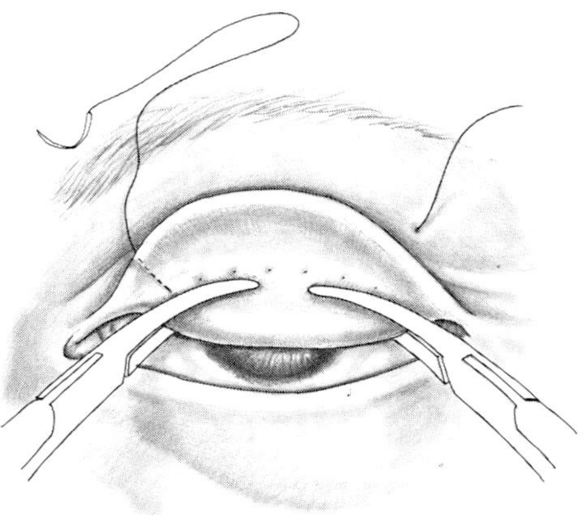

The tissue in front of the clamp is excised (Plate 13-5, *F*). The monofilament suture is tied on top of the lid. A light dressing is applied. The suture is removed after 1 week (Plate 13-5, *G*).

We have thus far had no problems with this technique. Since the needle enters and exits from the same site, no suture is exposed to the cornea on the underside of the lid.

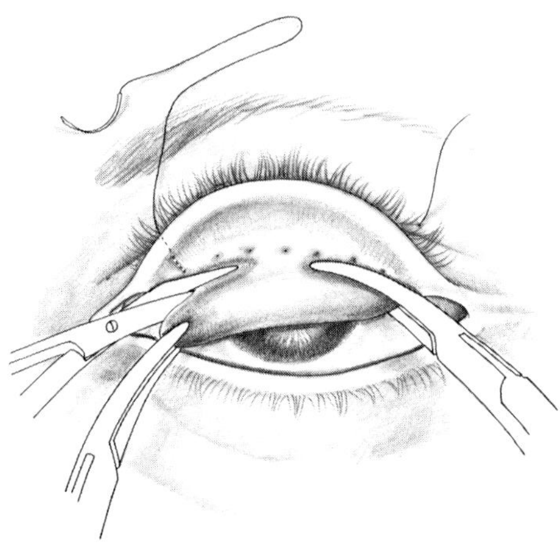

F, Resection of tissue in front of
clamp.

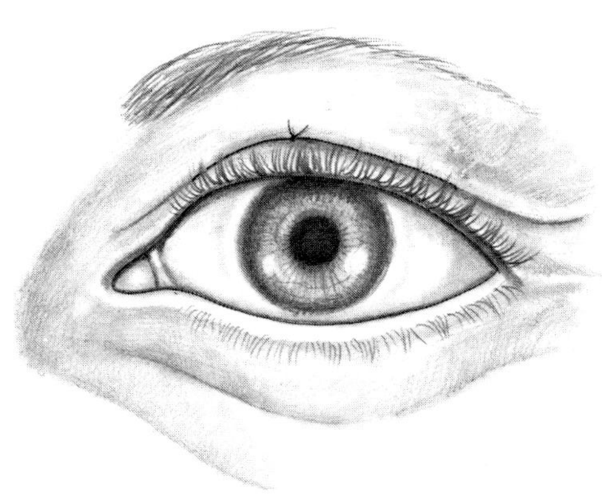

G, Suture tied in place.

PARALYTIC EYELID MALPOSITION

Paralysis of the seventh cranial nerve causes poor closure of the upper and lower eyelids. Generally, Bell's phenomenon will still elevate the cornea during an attempted blink and the levator muscle will relax with a slight lowering of the upper lid, but these actions will not adequately protect the cornea from desiccation and eventual ulceration and opacification.

The problem is first approached medically. Artificial tears, ocular lubricants, and ointments, together with patching during the evening and night, can frequently protect the cornea while the patient is observed for resolution of the seventh nerve palsy. However, a persistently increased lacrimal lake and epiphora from the failed tear pump will cause significant visual disturbances even if the cornea can be temporarily protected with this therapy. Therefore, medical therapy is only a temporizing treatment in this condition. Surgical therapy offers the only satisfactory intermediate and long-term solution.

Corneal exposure and compromise are helped by lateral tarsorrhaphy, which narrows the horizontal and vertical interpalpebral dimensions. The total surface area of the eye that must keep moist is thereby lessened. Tarsorrhaphy is relatively straightforward and can be done at the bedside under sterile conditions. It is also readily reversible.

The size of the tarsorrhaphy is determined by the severity of the patient's exposure keratopathy and the size of the original palpebral fissure. The greater the palpebral fissure and the exposure keratopathy, the larger the tarsorrhaphy. If it is necessary to occlude the visual axis to adequately protect the cornea, the surgeon should not hesitate to do so. There are many methods for closing the lid margin. Our preferred technique is presented below.

The most medial extent of the lateral tarsorrhaphy is marked on the upper and lower lids with a razor knife. The lid margin, above the lash line, is removed lateral to the mark and into the lateral canthus. A 5-0 Vicryl suture is passed into the skin near the lateral canthal angle and brought out through the newly created raw lid margin. It is brought out through the same raw lid margin, slightly more medially. The suture is passed repeatedly through the lid margin in a serpentine fashion until the medial edge of the tarsorrhaphy is reached. The suture is brought out through the skin edge. The lid margin is brought together by pulling on both ends of the suture (Plate 14-1, *A*). The suture is tied on itself at both points where it exits the skin.

A 4-0 silk mattress suture is placed through the anterior lamellae of the upper and lower lids. The suture is tied over rubber-band bolsters on the upper and lower lids (Plate 14-1, *B*). The eye is pressure patched with antibiotic ointment until the next day. The silk suture may be removed in 5 to 7 days and the Vicryl suture in 2 to 3 weeks. A tarsorrhaphy done in this manner can be reversed without significant cosmetic deformity.

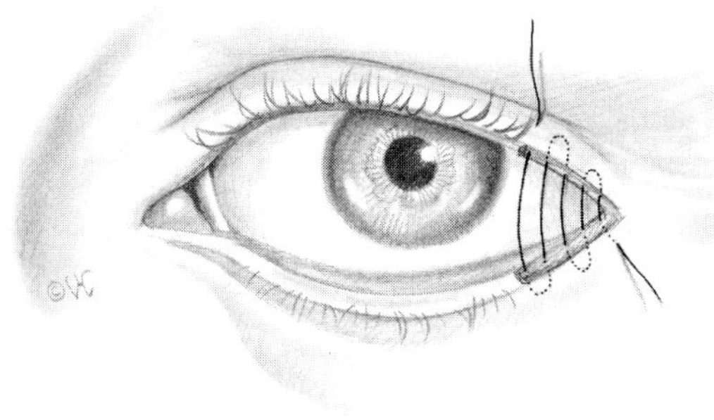

A, Serpentine suture used to close tarsorrhaphy site.

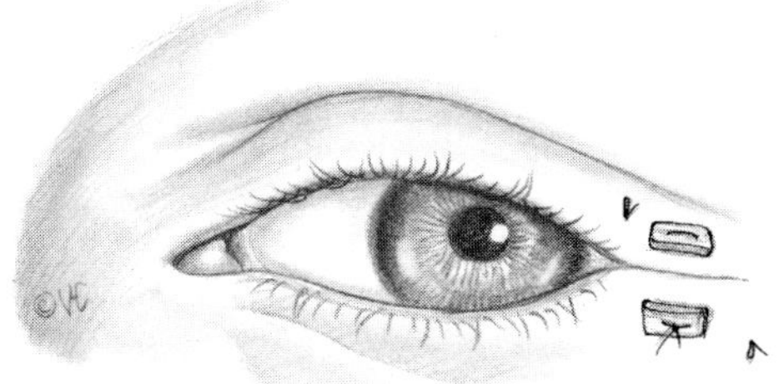

B, 6-0 silk suture tied over rubberband bolsters.

Several procedures have been described for the correction of paralytic upper eyelid malposition resulting from seventh nerve dysfunction. All of the procedures involve implantation of foreign material into the eyelids and are associated with early and late extrusion of this material. All of these procedures are complex and should be attempted only by surgeons experienced with implanting foreign material into the eyelids. We prefer implantation of a gold weight between the tarsus and the levator aponeurosis because of its effectiveness and the very low rate of extrusion.

The appropriate mass of the gold weight is determined by taping the weight to the lid and observing the patient in the upright position. The levator should be able to lift the weight attached to the eyelid, and the lid should close completely when the levator is relaxed.

The crease of the upper eyelid is marked with a marking pen. The lid is anesthetized by injecting a 50:50 mixture of 2% lidocaine and 0.75% Marcaine, both with 1:100,000 epinephrine, directly under the skin to avoid immobilizing the levator muscle. The lid is incised with a Bard-Parker or razor knife (Plate 14-2, *A*). A skin-muscle flap is then dissected inferiorly to the lash line, exposing the tarsus (Plate 14-2, *B*). The inferior edge of the orbital septum and the preorbital orbicularis just below the skin incision are grasped with Castroviejo forceps to place the septum on stretch. The septum is entered with curved iris scissors angled 45 degrees below the frontal plane and toward the crown of the head. The septum is opened medially and laterally. The preaponeurotic fat pad is seen between the levator aponeurosis and the septum.

Hemostasis is achieved with thermal cautery. The gold weight is placed anterior to the tarsus with two fixation holes on the upper side (Plate 14-2, *C*). The weight is sutured to the tarsus with 5-0 Novafil suture through all three fixation holes. Great care is taken to avoid full penetration of the tarsus with these sutures. The upper hole's suture is cut short. The lower two holes' sutures are kept long to attach levator aponeurosis to the tarsus, over the gold weight (Plate 14-2, *D*).

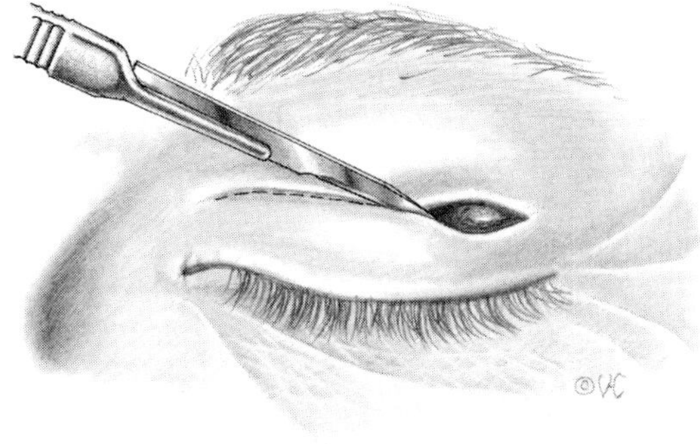

A, Lid incision made.

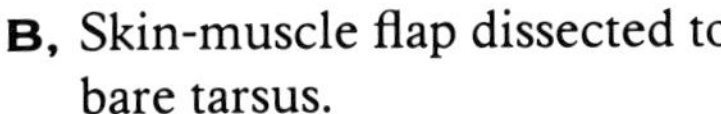

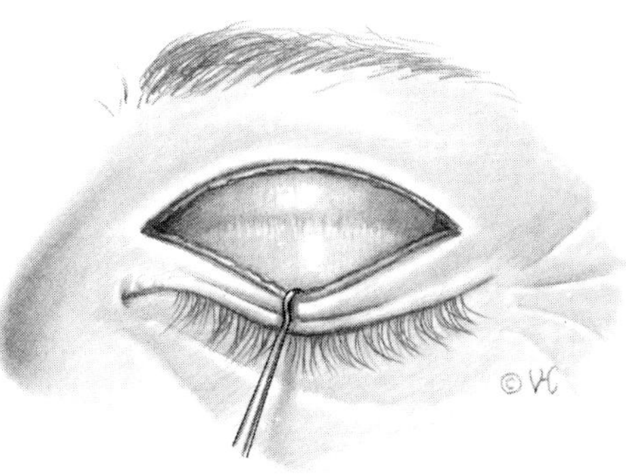

B, Skin-muscle flap dissected to bare tarsus.

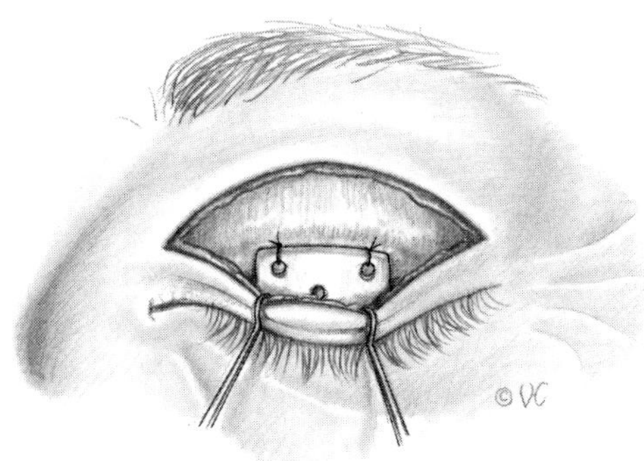

C, Gold weight sewn to tarsus with 5-0 Novafil sutures.

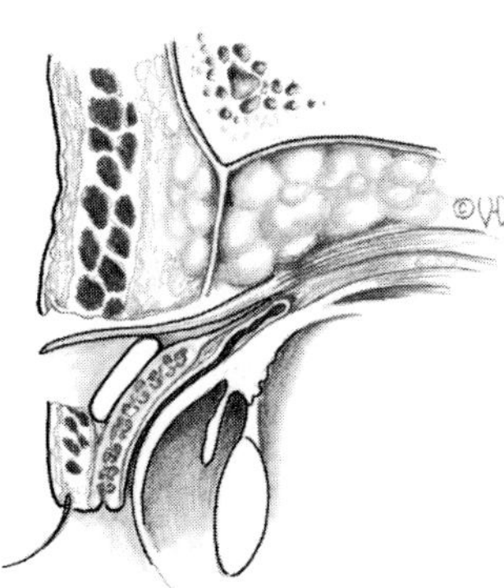

D, Sagittal view demonstrating levator over gold weight.

Advancing the levator complex over the gold weight and securing it with the two Novafil sutures may cause a significant lid retraction. The lid retraction is corrected by titrated, offset tenotomies of the aponeurosis, which will effectively lengthen the levator complex (Plate 14-2, *E* and *F*). The desired endpoint of the procedure is complete lid closure with a blink and an adequate opening of the lid while the patient is sitting upright on the surgical table. The gold weight is completely covered anteriorly with levator aponeurosis and posteriorly with tarsus. The orbicularis layer is closed with interrupted 5-0 Vicryl sutures. The skin is closed with interrupted 6-0 mild chromic sutures (Plate 14-2, *G*). The eye is pressure patched until the next morning. The patient is observed carefully in the postoperative period for corneal exposure and implant extrusion.

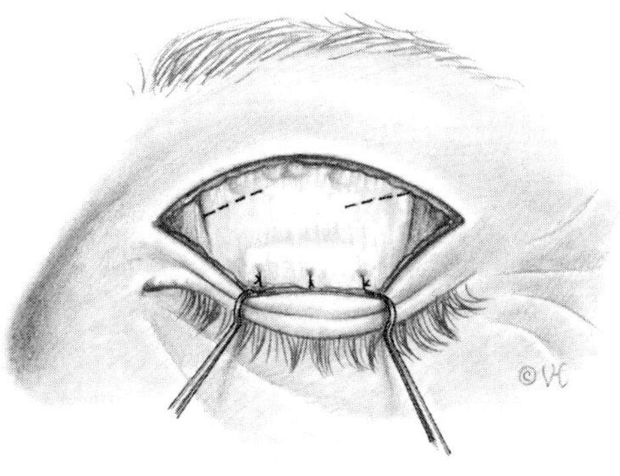

E, Tenotomy outlined in cases of overcorrected lid.

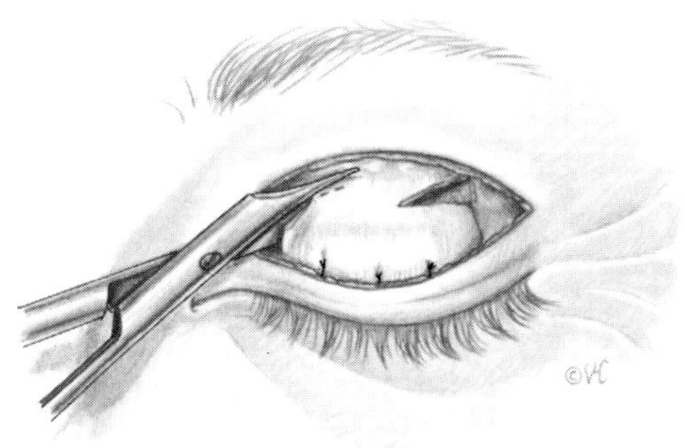

F, Tenotomy being completed.

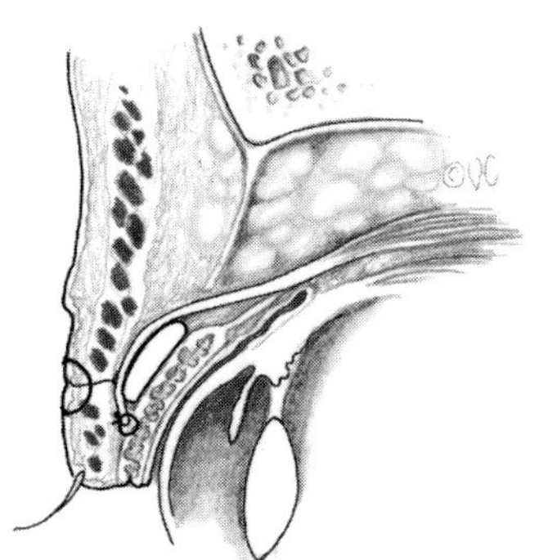

G, Incision site closed.

CHAPTER 15

SYMBLEPHARON

Progressive inflammatory disease such as pemphigoid and erythema multiforme, traumatic injuries, and chemical injuries tend to produce continual scarring and contracture of the conjunctiva, with destruction of all of its lubricating elements and a resultant entropion of both upper and lower lids. There is a gradual obliteration of the cul-de-sacs, and the resulting dryness causes corneal damage with opacity and vascularization of the cornea. Procedures such as Z-plasty, conjunctival transplantation, and the placement of scleral rings, while they may provide temporary relief, are eventually overcome by the unrelenting disease process. A procedure that we have used for these severe and desperate cases involves large mucous membrane grafts to re-form the cul-de-sacs and a lid-splitting technique as a cure for the entropion.

Because of the extensive dissection involved and the need for large buccal mucous membrane grafts to be taken, re-formation of cul-de-sacs is best performed with the patient under general anesthesia. Sutures of 6-0 silk are passed through the centers of the medial and temporal thirds of the upper and lower lid margins. The lids are maximally retracted.

A razor knife is used to dissect the scarred conjunctiva and free the lids from the adherent sclera (Plate 15-1, *A*). Profuse bleeding usually occurs. Continuous irrigation is most helpful during this dissection. The injection of local anesthetic with epinephrine is to no avail. Moderate pressure and vasoconstrictors are applied when the dissection is complete. Cautery should be avoided, since this is a graft bed. Lysis of the conjunctival bands is continued until the area of the recti insertions is reached. Care is taken not to damage these.

Split-thickness mucous membrane grafts are taken from the mouth, to be used as a lining for the cul-de-sacs. A Castroviejo mucotome set at 0.5 mm is used to obtain the donor grafts. The area from which the graft is to be taken is injected with 1% lidocaine with 1:100,000 epinephrine. In these cases it is usually necessary to utilize both upper and lower lids, as well as the mucosa of the cheeks. As each graft is taken, it is transferred to the recipient site, where it is meticulously sutured with 7-0 chromic catgut suture, the raw surface toward the globe (Plate 15-1, *B*).

The perilimbal area is sutured first. Because split-thickness grafts contract considerably, they should not be sutured in a stretched position. Finally, full-thickness 6-0 silk mattress sutures are placed in the fornices and tied over cotton bolsters on the external surfaces of the lids (Plate 15-1, *C*).

A scleral shell with the central area removed is placed over the globe, and the lids are sutured closed. The marginal sutures are removed after several days. However, the scleral shell is left in position until the graft has healed in place. Following an interval of 4 to 6 weeks, it is possible to attempt to repair the entropion.

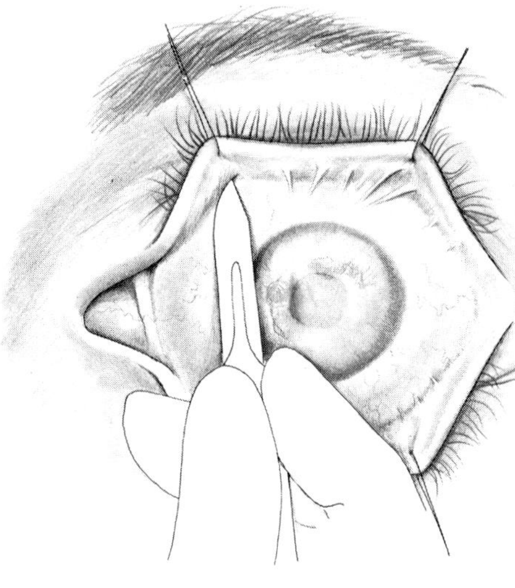

A, Adherent lids dissected from sclera.

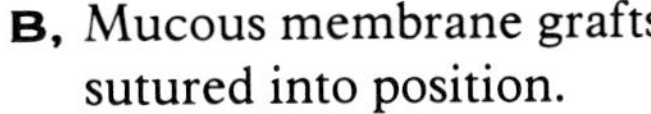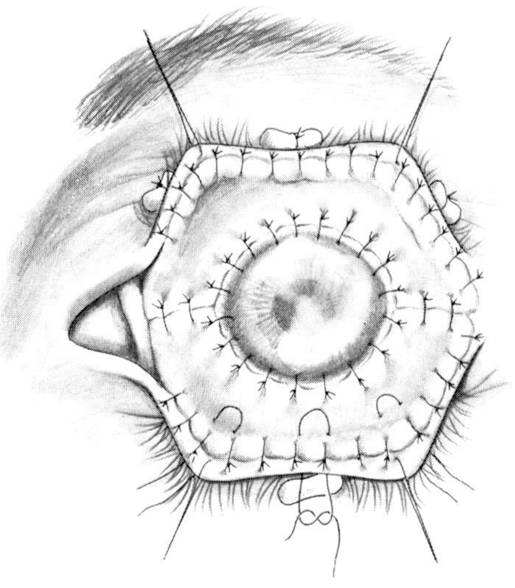

B, Mucous membrane grafts sutured into position.

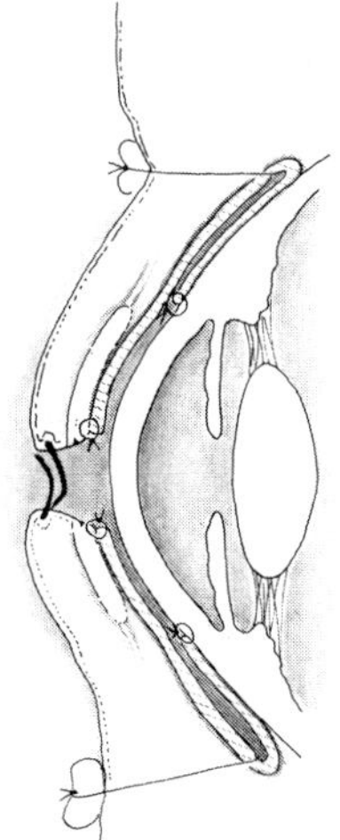

C, Sagittal section to illustrate placement of sutures in cul-de-sacs.

A razor knife is used to make an incision at the mucocutaneous junction of the upper and lower lids, splitting the lids into two lamellae. The incision is carried laterally from an area temporal to the punctum almost to the lateral canthus (Plate 15-2, *A*).

The dissection is continued deep enough into each lid that 5 mm of posterior lamella can be advanced. The advanced lamellae are sutured together with continuous 5-0 chromic catgut. The lid margins are recessed and sutured to the upper portion of the advanced lamellae with interrupted 6-0 chromic sutures (Plate 15-2, *B* and *C*).

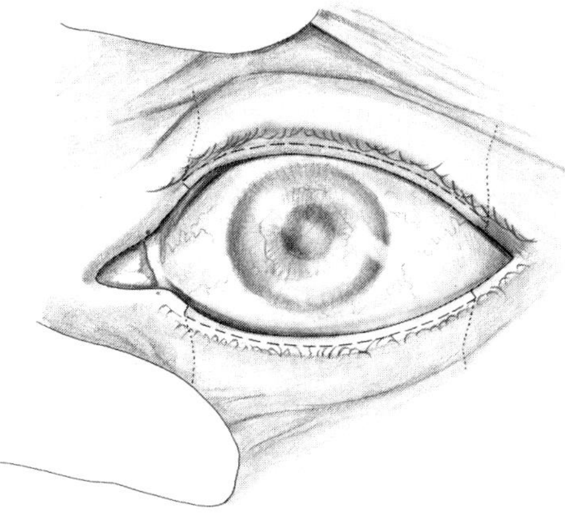

A, Horizontal midmarginal tarsal incision and external incisions outlined.

B, Internal lamellae advanced and sutured into place.

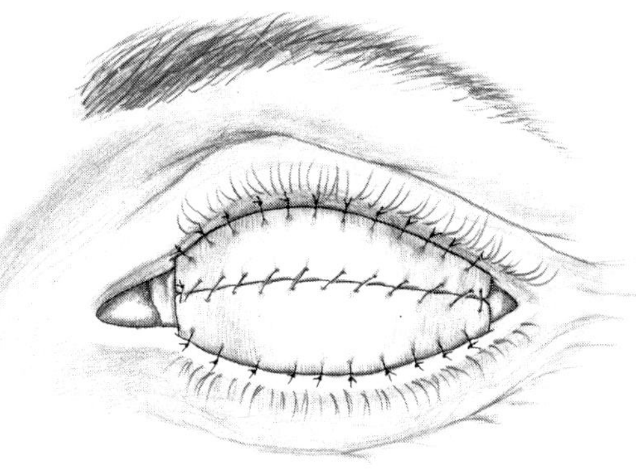

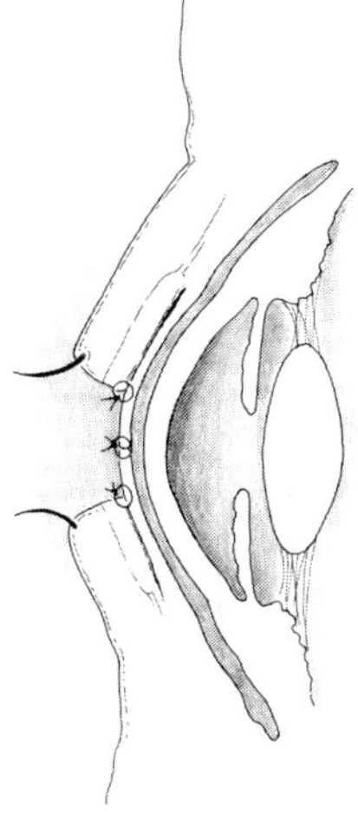

C, Sagittal view to illustrate advancement and suturing of internal lamallae. Note recession of lid margins.

A full-thickness (1 mm) mucous membrane graft is obtained freehand from the area of the lower lip to fit over the area created by the posterior lamellae. This is sutured into place with interrupted 6-0 chromic catgut sutures (Plate 15-2, *D*). After a period of 2 months, to allow for healing and detumescence of the tissue, the graft is opened. The lid margins regress and hypertrophy over several months (Plate 15-2, *E*).

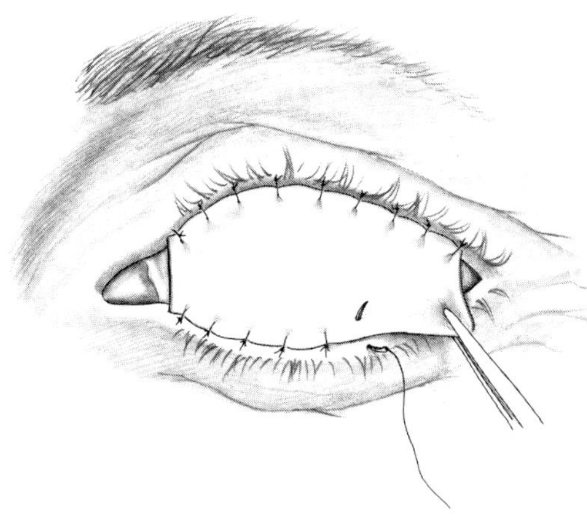

D, Full-thickness mucous membrane graft sutured into place.

E, Tarsorrhaphy opened after 8 weeks.

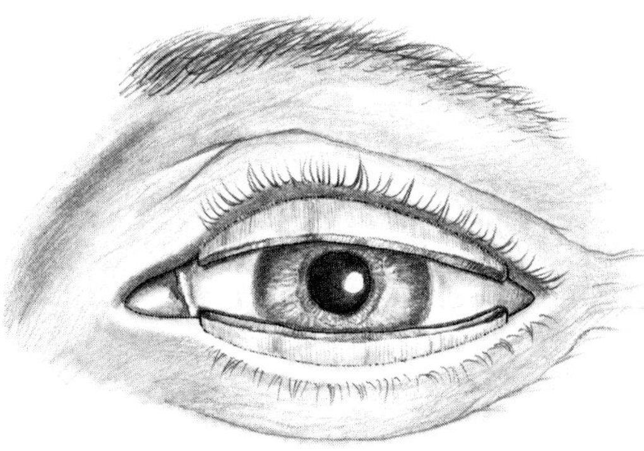

RECURRENT PTERYGIA

The treatment for recurrent or hypertrophic pterygia, once it has been ascertained that one is dealing with a benign condition, is the adequate resection of the involved tissue and the placement of normal tissue in the area to act as an anatomic barrier.

Following the injection of a local anesthetic into the lids by the modified Van Lint method, a lid speculum is placed into position to provide adequate exposure of the globe. The pterygium is gently grasped with fixation forceps, and a solution of 1% lidocaine with 1:100,000 epinephrine is injected into the tissue superficial to the corneal stroma. This not only provides akinesia but also facilitates dissection (Plate 16-1, *A*).

With a razor knife, dissection is initiated at the apex of the lesion. A superficial keratectomy is performed, and the pterygium is dissected back over the limbus and onto the episclera (Plate 16-1, *B*). With the pterygium stretched, the dissection is carried to the insertion of the medial rectus muscle. All involved tissue is then resected, with care taken not to injure the muscle insertion.

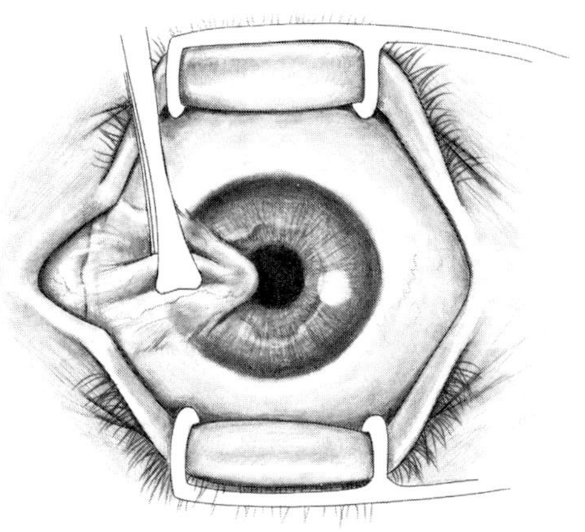

A, Pterygium occupying nasal aspect of cornea.

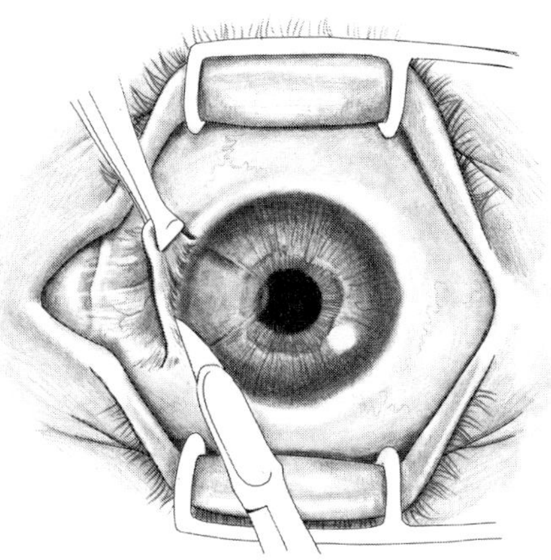

B, Dissection of pterygium from cornea and sclera.

A crescent incision is made about 1 mm from the limbus from the 12 o'clock to the 6 o'clock position. A second, concentric incision is created 5 mm temporal to this (Plate 16-1, *C*). The flap is left attached at each extremity, but it is dissected free in the central portion.

The recipient bed should be carefully cleaned of any fibrotic material. Hemostasis is achieved by applying pressure and by vasoconstrictors, as in any graft bed.

The conjunctival flap is then carefully transposed to the new site. Sutures of 7-0 chromic catgut are placed to orient the flap in several areas. This accomplished, meticulous suturing should continue until the flap is evenly secured in place. The bases of the flap are not sutured, because any redundant tissue here will flatten over a several-week period (Plate 16-1, *D*).

The donor site is likewise closed with interrupted sutures of 7-0 chromic catgut. The site will generally close with minimal tension. However, a scleral hook is useful in bringing together the ends of the tissue during suturing (Plate 16-1, *E*).

A light dressing is applied and is changed daily for several days. No ointment is used. In the postoperative period the transplanted area vascularizes along the arc of the graft. This inhibits horizontal regrowth of the pterygium.

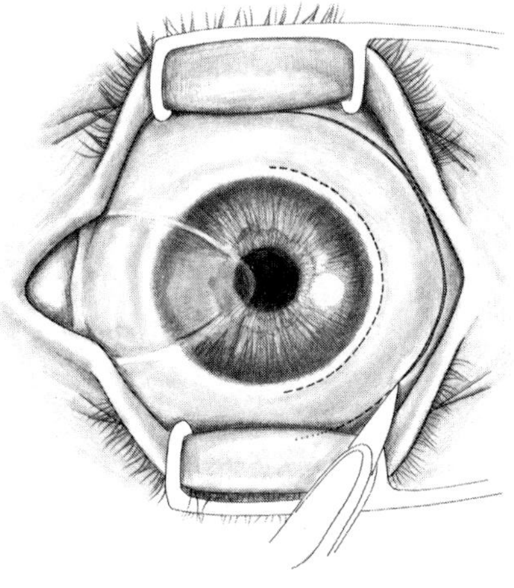

C, Conjunctival flap prepared.

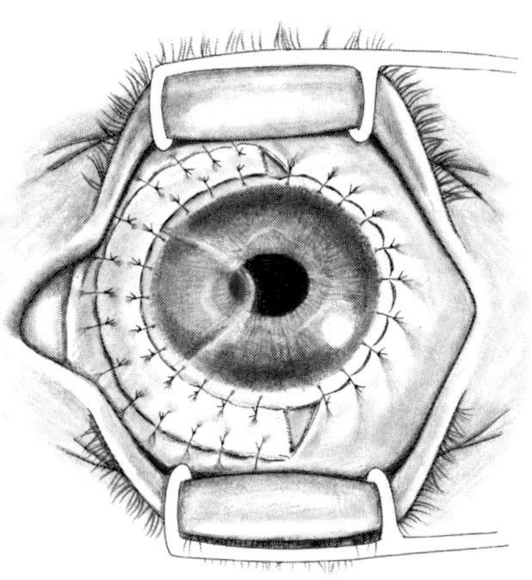

D, Conjunctival flap transposed and sutured into place.

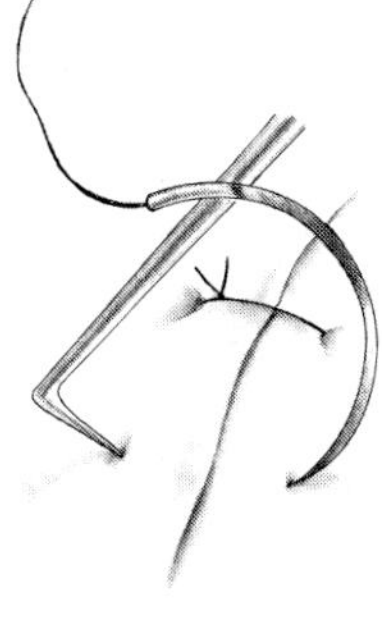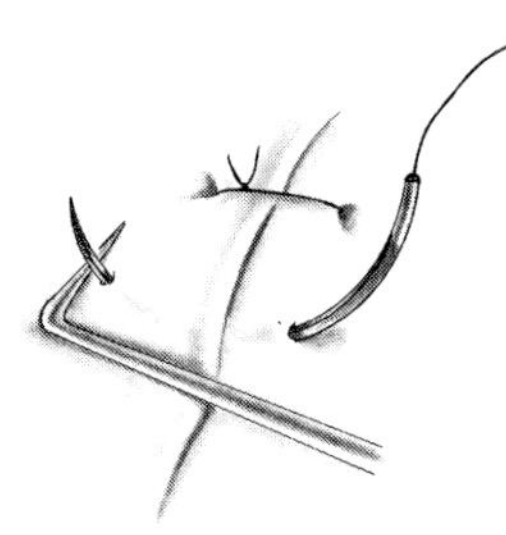

E, Scleral hook used during suture insertion.

SOCKET RECONSTRUCTION

In those cases in which contracture of tissues in the anophthalmic socket has made even the most skillful fitting of a prosthetic device an impossibility, the surgeon must replace the deficiency of tissue with a suitable substitute. Commonly seen in cases involving inflammatory disease, traumatic injury, tissue avulsion, chemical burns, or faulty enucleation technique or following involutional fibrotic change, a contracted socket results from a shortening or shrinkage of the tissue in the orbit.

The surgeon has several choices for repairing the defect. Mucous membrane grafts can be used in cases in which the contracture is mild and limited. The techniques of taking these grafts and inserting them will be described. For more extensive cases a split-thickness skin graft can be used to line the entire socket.

In some cases the original implant will have extruded or migrated. In these cases we have successfully used a composite dermis-fat graft not only to replace the implant but also to increase the dimension of the socket.

General anesthesia is preferred for mucous membrane grafts.

Following the placement of 6-0 silk sutures at the centers of the medial and temporal thirds of the upper and lower lids to act as traction sutures, a Bard-Parker blade is used to horizontally incise the contracted conjunctival tissue (Plate 17-1, *A*). The injection of a local anesthetic with epinephrine is of limited value in achieving hemostasis but in some cases does aid in hydraulic dissection.

Sharp scissors are used to undermine the conjunctival tissue. It is useful to grasp the tissue edges with skin hooks and exert traction in the opposite direction of the dissection. The conjuctiva is dissected inferiorly first and then superiorly to the lid margin. Special care is taken in the upper lid dissection not to injure the upper lid retractors (Plate 17-1, *B*).

A horizontal incision is then made over the inferior orbital rim. The incision should be made full thickness down to the bone. The rim is palpated and can be used as a guide and support. A hemostat is used to spread the surrounding tissue and allow good exposure of the bony rim. A drilling device is then used to create a full-thickness hole in the inferior orbital rim (Plate 17-1, *B*).

With skin hooks used to retract the conjunctival lining, the subconjunctival fibrotic tissue in the socket should be excised to allow placement of a conformer. Once again, any dissection in the superior cul-de-sac should be done with care to avoid disrupting the levator muscle or its aponeurosis. The inferior dissection should be as close as possible to the hole drilled through the inferior orbital rim (Plate 17-1, *C*).

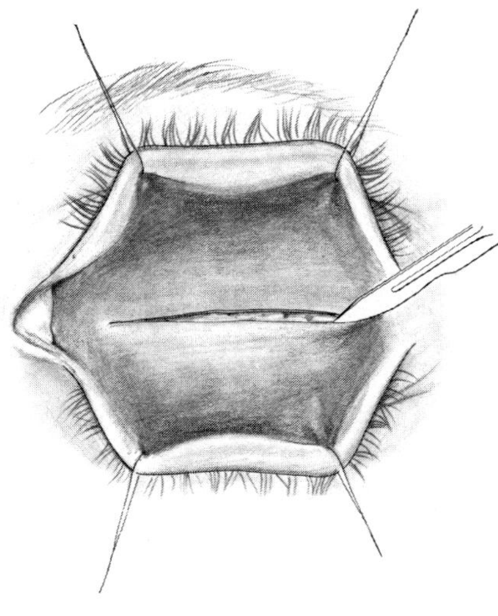

A, Lids retracted and horizontal incision made.

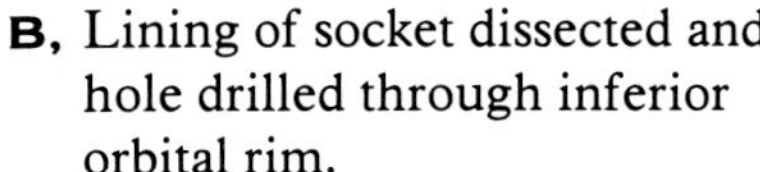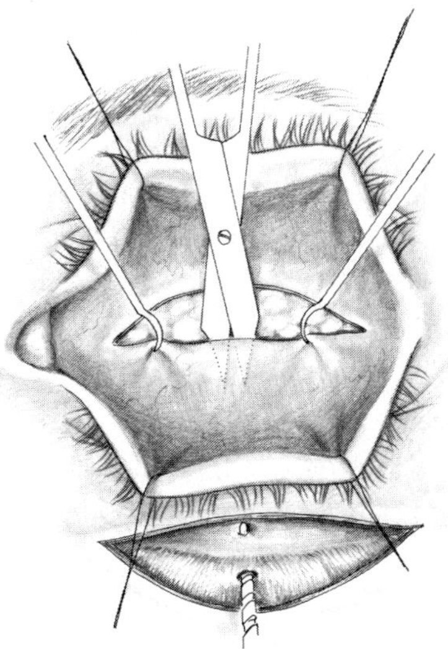

B, Lining of socket dissected and hole drilled through inferior orbital rim.

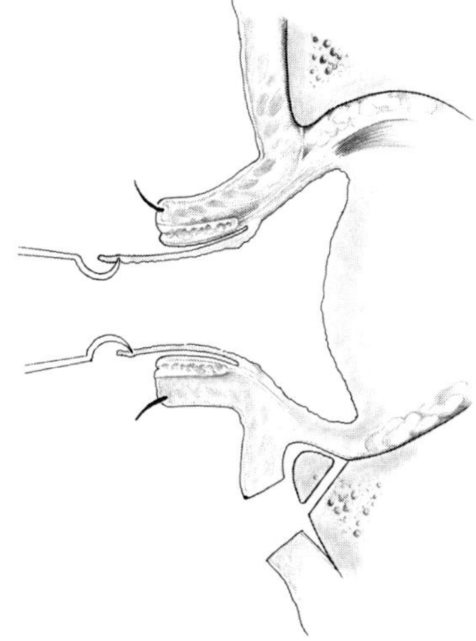

C, Sagittal view of new socket

A conformer is then molded to the socket. The material we prefer is dental molding compound, which can be softened in warm water and molded with no great difficulty in the operating room. The edges of the conformer should be smooth and the center drilled out so that an 8- to 10-mm opening is present to facilitate fluid drainage.

In the inferior portion of the doughnut-shaped conformer, another smaller hole should be drilled, which will come into proximity with the hole drilled in the inferior orbital rim.

The mucous membrane graft should be relatively thick (0.8 mm). The lower lip is everted and held in position with an appropriate clamp or towel hooks. The mucosa is injected with 1% lidocaine with 1:100,000 epinephrine. In these areas the surgeon uses a razor knife instead of a mucotome to take a freehand graft, so that he is certain to obtain a reasonably thick graft. Split-thickness grafts will contract up to 50%. The donor site need not be sutured, but will freely granulate.

The mucous membrane is folded over the conformer with the raw surface outward (Plate 17-1, *D*). It is then placed in the dissected cavity so that the raw surface is in contact with the newly dissected area. The mucous membrane graft is sutured with moderate tension to the conformer lining with absorbable suture. The conformer is then removed and perforated at the center for drainage.

If the area to be re-formed is large, split-thickness skin from a smooth area of the body is obtained with a mechanical dermatome. It is used in a similar fashion.

A fine stainless steel wire is then threaded through the hole in the inferior orbital rim and passed through the socket and out between the lids. The wire is passed through the graft and the smaller inferior hole in the conformer. The conformer is threaded into place in the socket. The wire is then secured in place by being twisted with a hemostat, and it is brought into apposition with the inferior orbital rim. The end is clipped with a wire cutter and rotated to remain within the conformer.

The incision overlying the inferior orbital rim is closed in layered fashion, with 5-0 chromic catgut used to close the subcutaneous layer and interrupted sutures of 6-0 silk used to close the skin (Plate 17-1, *E*).

Interpalpebral sutures of 6-0 silk are placed, which together with the stainless steel wire will hold the conformer in place (Plate 17-1, *F*).

The skin and interpalpebral sutures are removed after 4 days. A light dressing is changed daily for several days. Postoperatively, topical antibiotics are used.

The conformer is left in place for approximately 4 to 6 weeks, at which time the wire is cut and the conformer removed. A temporary conformer is placed in position until a prosthetic device can be fitted.

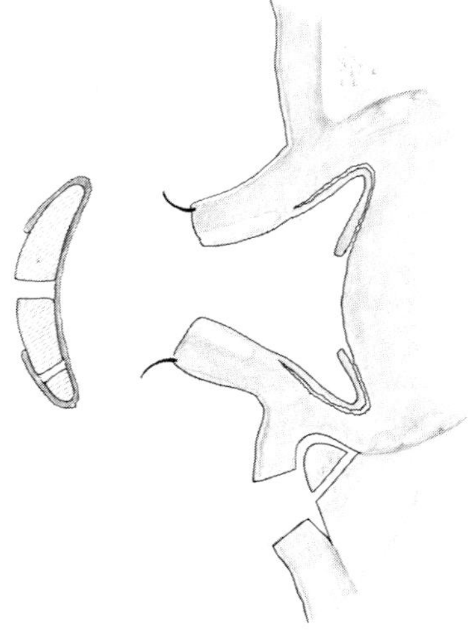

D, Conformer shaped to fit new socket and conformer lined with mucous membrane.

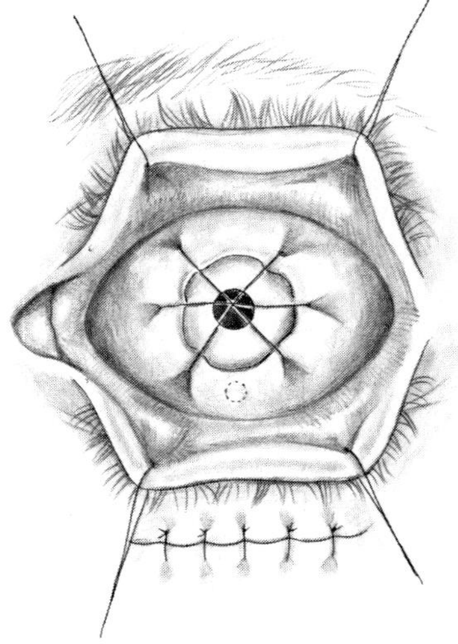

E, Conformer sutured into place and skin incision closed.

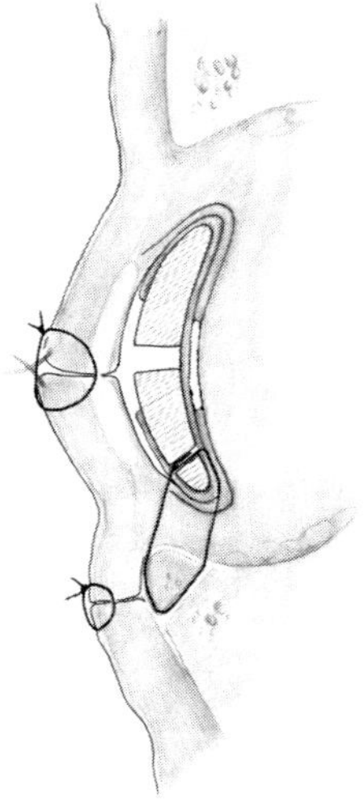

F, Sagittal view to illustrate conformer wired into position.

The use of autogenous dermis-fat grafts as a replacement for migrated or extruding orbital implants has proven to be an excellent method for secondary replacement of these primary synthetic implants.

A variety of materials have been used for orbital implants: sclera, fascia lata, and temporal fascia. The extrusion or migration of orbital implants is a common complication of enucleation. Not only does it produce a cosmetic defect, but also the recurrent exposure and infection of tissue cause a contraction of the socket. The added benefit of dermis-fat grafting is an increase in the dimension of the socket.

When the patient has a migrated and/or partially extruding orbital implant, one is generally able to palpate the implant through the closed lid to ascertain its location (Plate 17-2, *A*). This should be done preoperatively and noted. Later, with the patient in the supine position in the operating room, this is more difficult.

General anesthesia is required for this procedure. A lid speculum (or 6-0 silk traction sutures) is placed in the eye to give adequate exposure. If the implant is extruding, the area of conjunctival erosion is visible (Plate 17-2, *B*). We generally enter from this area and extend the incision from here.

Dissection is carried down through Tenon's capsule into the area in which the implant lies. The implant is isolated and removed. If the implant is not within the central cavity, an attempt is made to locate it (Plate 17-2, *C*).

After removal of the implant, an attempt is made to locate the muscle stumps that have retracted into the orbit. Forceps are inserted into the sheath in which the muscles lie, and after the stumps have been located they are grasped with hemostats (Plate 17-2, *D*).

Sutures of 4-0 chromic catgut are then passed through the rectus muscles at the 12, 3, 6, and 9 o'clock positions (Plate 17-2, *E*).

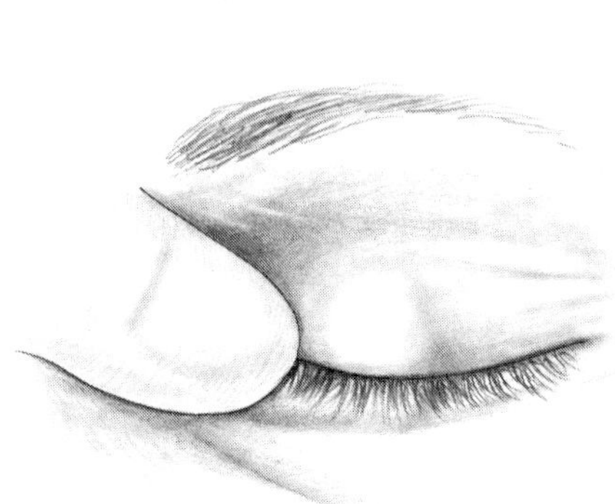

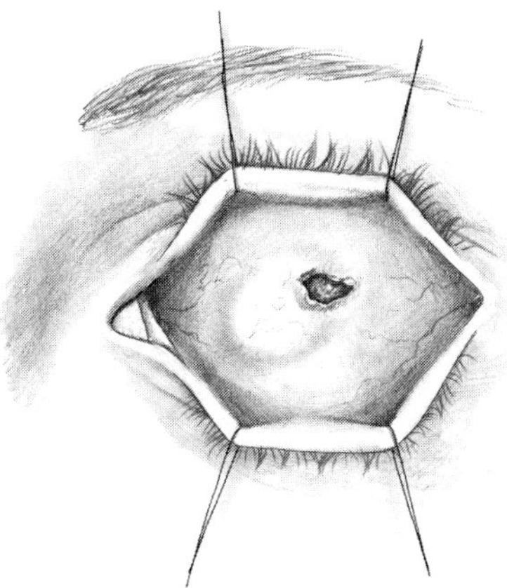

A, Position of extruding or migrating implant palpated through lid.

B, Implant extruding through conjunctiva.

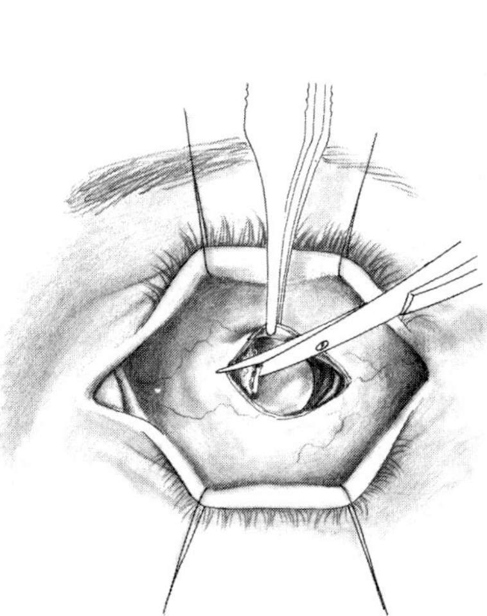

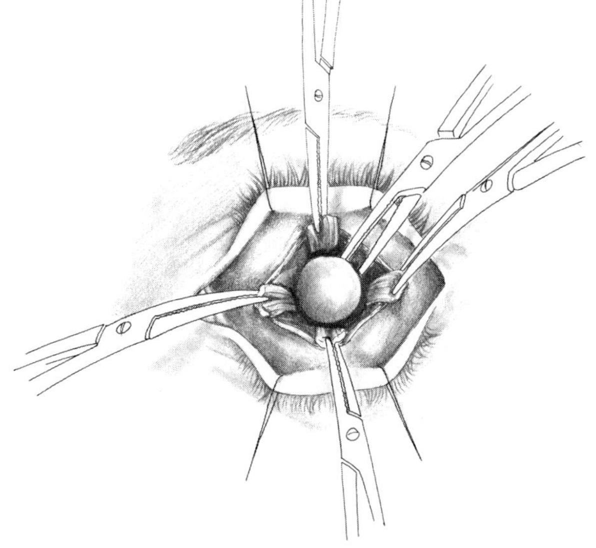

C, Dissection extended down to isolate implant.

D, Area of horizontal rectus muscles grasped and implant removed.

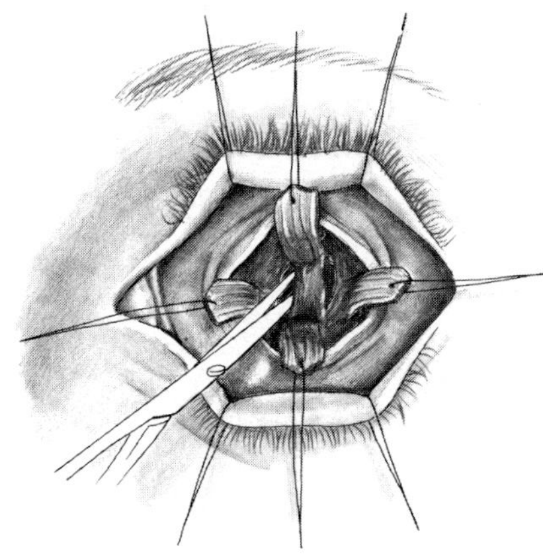

E, Sutures passed through muscle stumps.

Next, attention is turned to the lateral aspect of the thigh near the buttocks, which is prepared and marked for incision (Plate 17-2, *F*). A handheld dermabrader is used to abrade and deepithelialize an area of about 8 by 10 cm. The end point is reached when active bleeding occurs (Plate 17-2, *G*).

The graft is fashioned with a Bard-Parker blade to fit the size of the defect to be filled. Generally, a circumference of about 1.5 cm is sufficient. Because this area of the body has an abundant amount of subcutaneous fat, it is not difficult to remove about 4 cm of fat with the dermis (Plate 17-2, *H*).

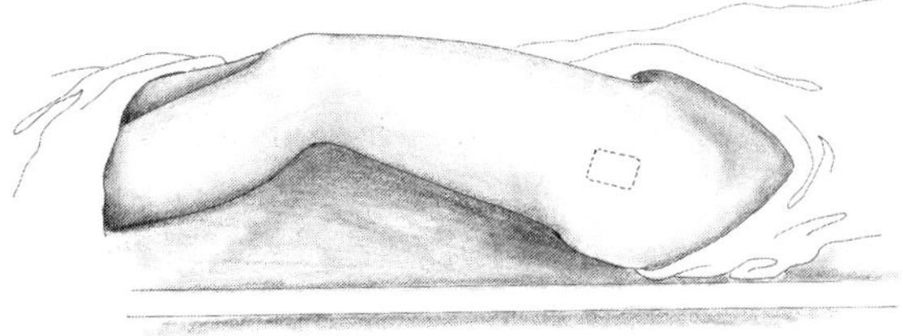

F, Area from which dermis-fat graft is to be taken.

G, Area deepithelialized with handheld dermabrader.

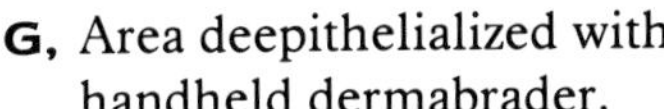

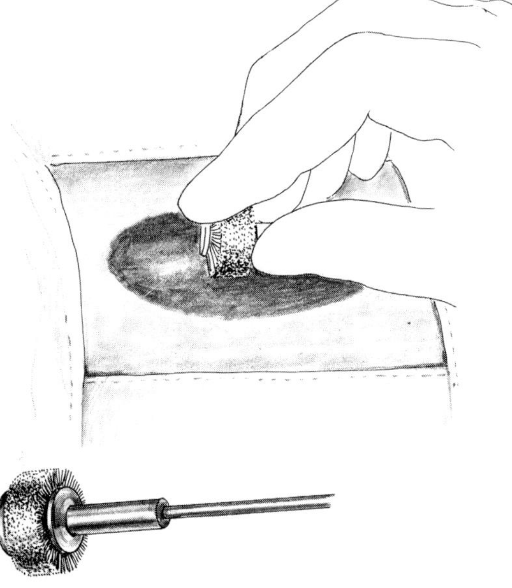

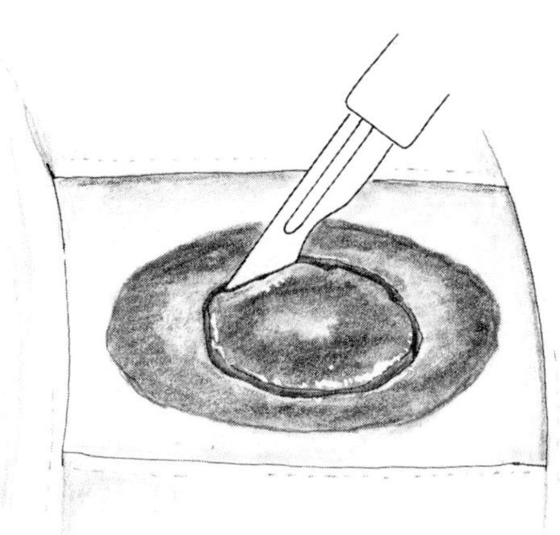

H, Dermis-fat graft excised.

We generally close the donor site in a layered fashion with buried sutures of 4-0 Vicryl-mic catgut and interrupted superficial sutures of 5-0 silk (Plate 17-2, *I*). The silk sutures are removed after 1 week, and the area reepithelializes in about a month. It is also possible to use near-far, far-near sutures to close the defect, because this two-layered closure will eliminate dead space.

The dermis-fat graft is gently transferred to the recipient bed. No irrigation is used in inserting the graft (Plate 17-2, *J*).

The 4-0 chromic sutures holding the rectus muscles are then sutured directly to the dermis. These four critical sutures hold the graft in place (Plate 17-2, *K*). Some fat may prolapse from the graft edges, but this can be excised later.

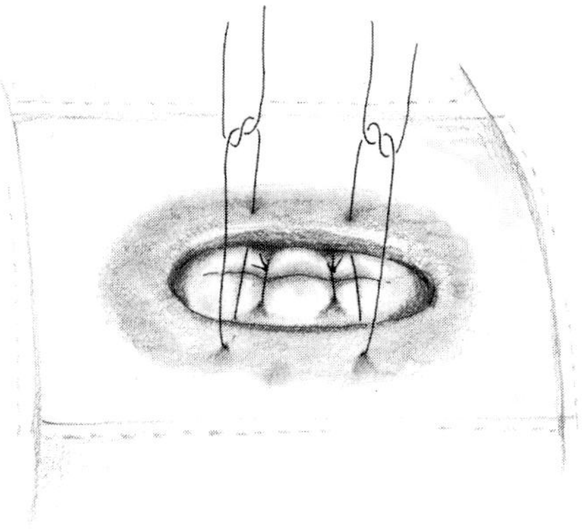

I, Donor site closed.

J, Dermis-fat graft to be transferred to socket.

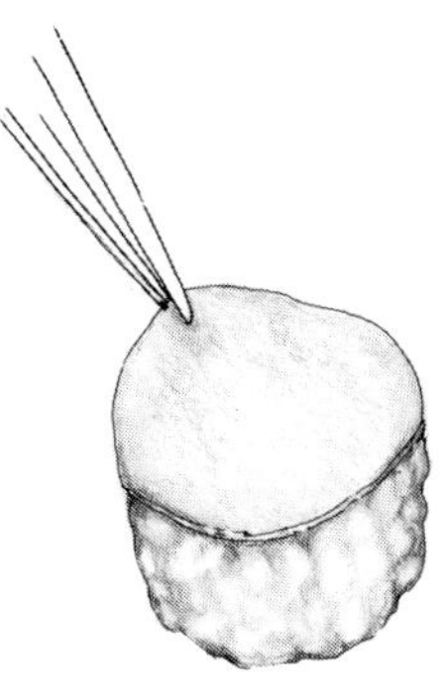

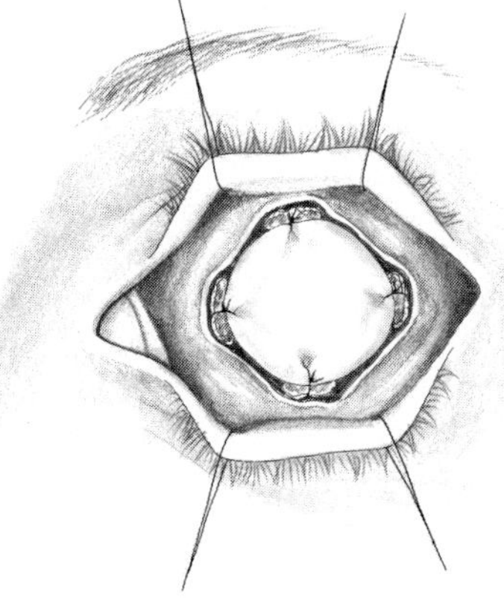

K, Graft first sutured to horizontal rectus muscles.

Additional 4-0 chromic sutures are then placed in interrupted fashion in each quadrant while the rectus sutures at the extremity of the quadrant are stretched (Plate 17-2, *L*).

The four quadrants are then successively closed (Plate 17-2, *M*). Closing the wound without use of the traction method is unnecessarily cumbersome.

The dermis is sutured directly to the conjunctiva and Tenon's capsule so that the graft at the completion of the suturing resembles a corneal button sewn into place (Plate 17-2, *N*).

A doughnut-shaped conformer is then placed in the socket, where it remains until a prosthetic eye is fitted in 4 to 6 weeks. The conjunctival epithelium grows over the graft in 1 month (Plate 17-2, *O*).

A light dressing is applied and changed daily for several days. Postoperatively, antibiotic drops are instilled for several weeks.

The motility obtained with this method is excellent, and recently we have used it as a primary procedure in a limited number of cases.

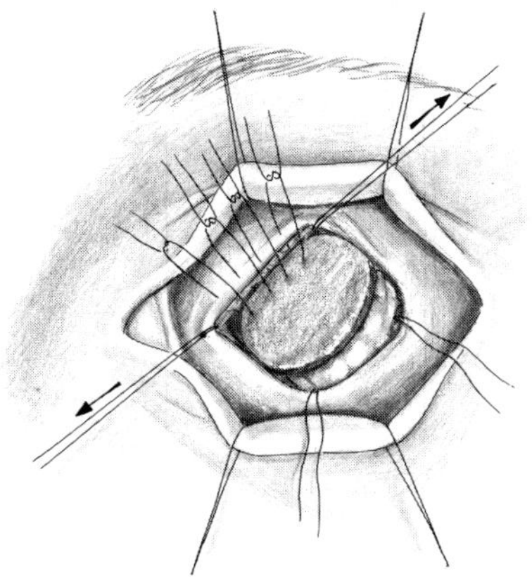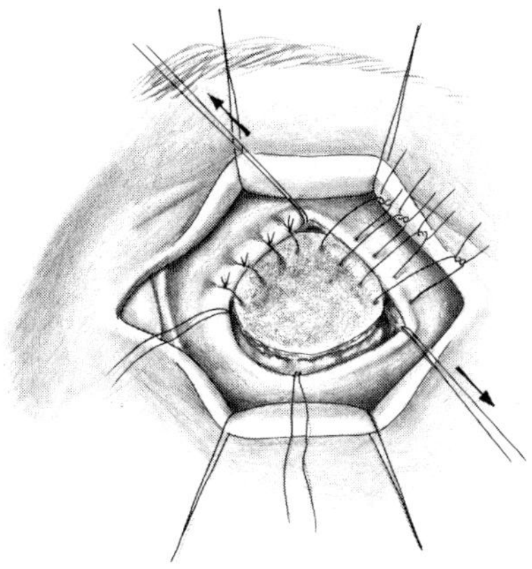

L and **M,** interrupted sutures used to complete closure as illustrated.

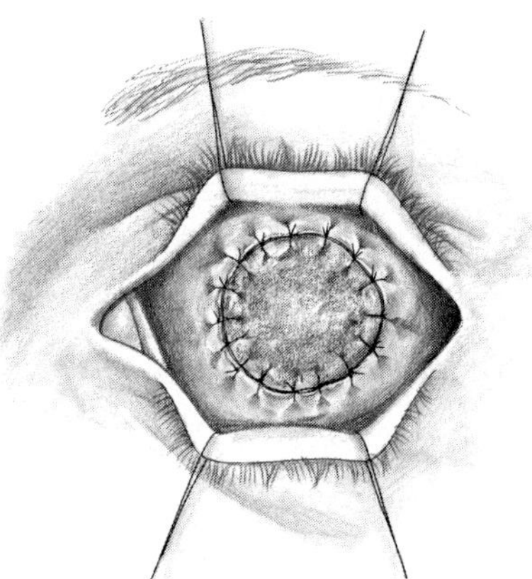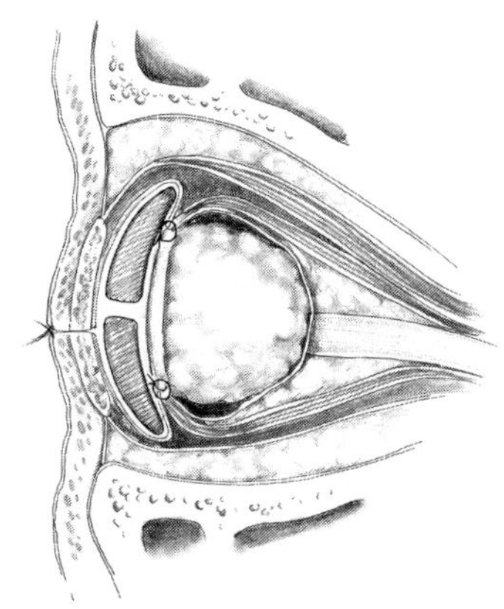

N, Donor graft sutures in place.

O, Sagittal view with conformer in place.

CHAPTER 18

ORBITAL FRACTURES AND MEDIAL CANTHAL RECONSTRUCTION

Orbital fractures can generally be divided into two broad categories: blow-out fractures of the orbital floor (or walls) and fractures involving the orbital rim. Included in the latter category are naso-orbital fractures.

An external force striking the orbital rim meets the strong bony abutment of the orbital region, which generally protects the orbit and its contents from significant damage (Plate 18-1, *A*). However, if the impact of the force is on the lids and globe, the orbital contents are retropulsed, with a sudden increase in intraorbital pressure and as a result the thin portion of the orbital floor or medial wall or both are fractured (Plate 18-1, *B*). This is a blow-out fracture of the orbit. These fractures are usually caused by blunt objects. Fractures of the orbital rim may also occur, in which case both entities must be treated.

Some cases may be very complicated. The orbital floor has been fractured and the contents of the orbit, bone fragments, and tissue adjacent to the inferior oblique and inferior rectus muscles have prolapsed into the maxillary sinus. In other cases, the damage is not as extensive and symptoms are caused by swelling around these tissues, which may restrict movement of the muscles.

Functionally, the vertical muscle imbalance secondary to the swelling or entrapment of the tissues near the inferior rectus or inferior oblique muscle is the greatest problem. Enophthalmos caused by the prolapse of tissue from the orbital cavity or enlargement of the cavity itself is also a frequent problem. The diplopia that occurs secondary to the vertical muscle imbalance ceases with the restoration of proper ocular movement. One must keep in mind the possibility of direct injury to the motor nerve supply or to the muscles themselves as a cause for delayed resolution of symptoms.

Generally, blow-out fractures cause little damage to the globe itself. If visual loss occurs and slit-lamp and funduscopic examinations have shown normal results, one must check for hemorrhage, edema, or fracture at the orbital apex or occlusion of the vascular supply to the optic nerve or retina. The area supplied by the infraorbital nerve often has lost sensation. A forced duction test should be performed, although a positive result may only signify the presence of edema, hemorrhage, or fat entrapment.

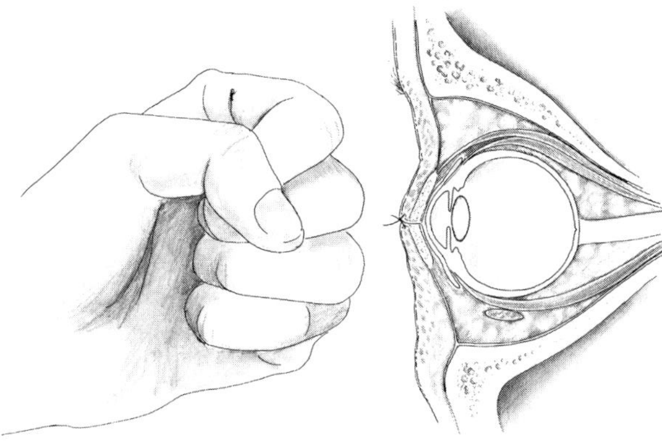

A, External force about to strike orbital area.

B, Increase in intraorbital pressure causes fracture of orbital floor.

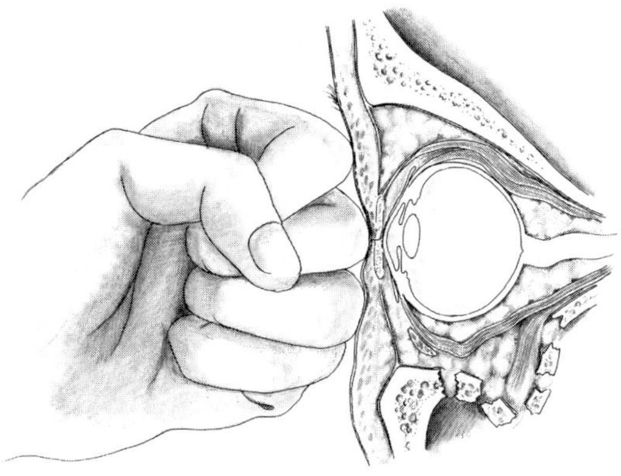

Orbital fractures need to be repaired if they cause significant enophthalmos or diplopia. They also need to be repaired if greater than 50% of the orbital floor is involved. The best method of reducing the orbital blow-out fracture is through a subciliary incision (Plate 18-2, *A*), although a cul-de-sac approach is an option (Plate 18-2, *B*). Polymethylmethacrelate mesh is used to cover the fracture site after the herniated tissue is reduced.

General anesthesia is preferred to intravenous sedation. The inferior lid and lateral canthus are infiltrated with 1% lidocaine with 1:100,000 epinephrine for hemostasis. The subciliary incision is made through skin into orbicularis with a razor knife from just below the puncta laterally to the canthal angle and extended several millimeters into a smile crease. The suborbicularis space is entered laterally with iris scissors. Blunt dissection is extended medially with a small curved hemostat. The remaining bridge of orbicularis is severed with curved iris scissors. The myocutaneous flap is retracted inferiorly with a Desmarres retractor (Plate 18-2, *C*). Hemostasis is achieved with thermal cautery.

The inferior orbital rim is identified. A piece of cotton gauze is placed over the index finger and rubbed vigorously over the inferior orbital rim and just below it to minimize blood flow to the area. A maleable retractor is placed against the orbital septum just lateral to the lower lid punctum and pressed against the inferior orbital floor. The periosteum just anterior and inferior to the orbital rim is incised with a no. 15 Bard-Parker blade from just below the punctum to just medial of the canthus. The maleable retractor is rotated with the scapel to protect the globe.

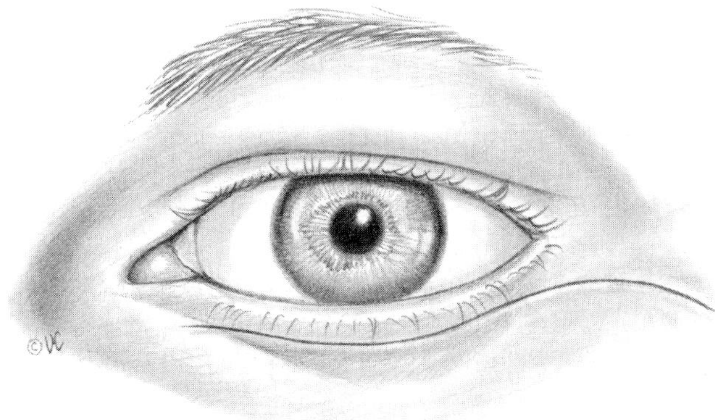

A, Subciliary incision designated.

B, Optional cul-de-sac approach.

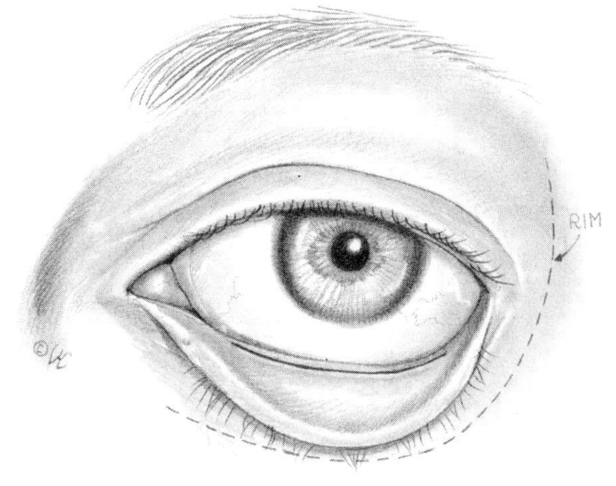

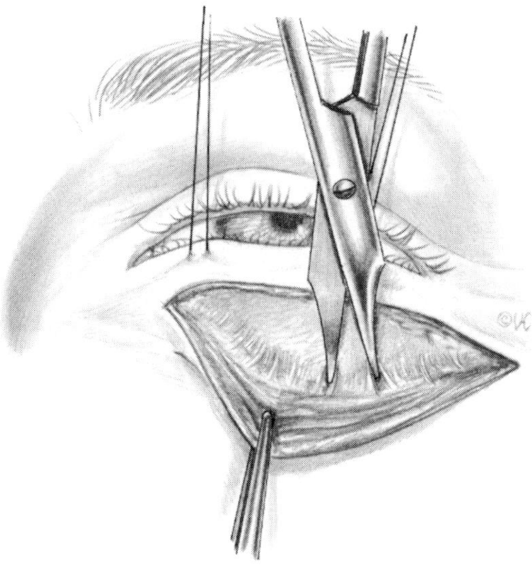

C, Orbital rim exposed with sharp dissection.

The periosteum is elevated posteriorly over the orbital rim, and the orbital floor is explored. The fracture is identified (Plate 18-2, *D*). It is reduced by using the periosteal elevator and the metal suction tip to reposit the herniated orbital tissue without tearing it. The two instruments are used alternatingly to hold and pull the tissue being reduced. The eye must be given regular periods of no manipulation and no external pressure every 5 to 10 minutes. If necessary, a rongeur can be used to aid in reduction (Plate 18-2, *E*).

After all of the material has been returned to the orbit, the fracture site is covered with polymethylmethacrelate mesh or other suitable material (Plate 18-2, *F*) to prevent any recurrent herniation. The mesh does not need to be fixated. It will not migrate and will not be perceptible to the patient.

Periosteum is closed with interrupted 5-0 Vicryl sutures. The orbicularis is not closed with sutures. The skin is closed with interrupted 6-0 mild chromic sutures. The eye is pressure patched with steroid and antibiotic ointment for approximately 30 minutes, and then the pressure patch is removed. The exact time the patch is to be removed is written directly on it to ensure the nursing staff will remove the patch in the appropriate time frame. Cold compresses are placed on the eye in the recovery room and at home for the first postoperative day or two.

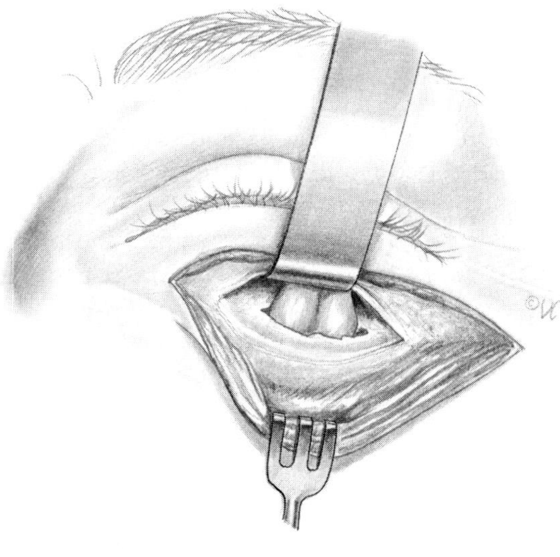

D, Myocutaneous flap retracted, periosteum incised, and orbital floor fracture site identified.

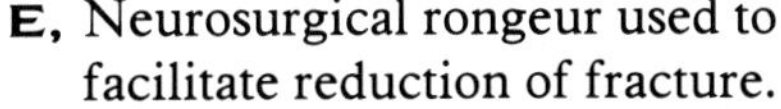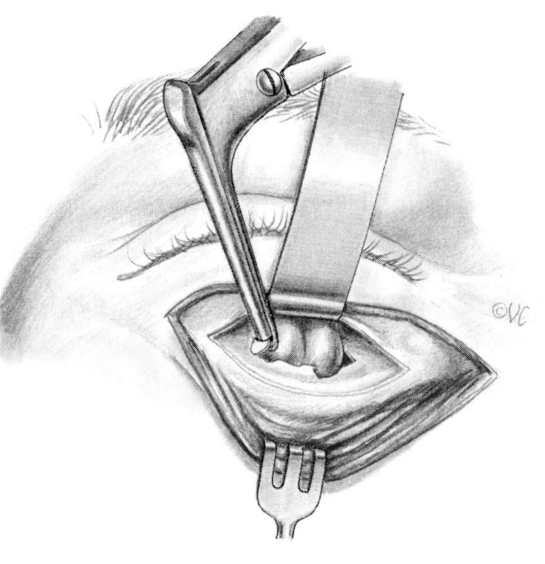

E, Neurosurgical rongeur used to facilitate reduction of fracture.

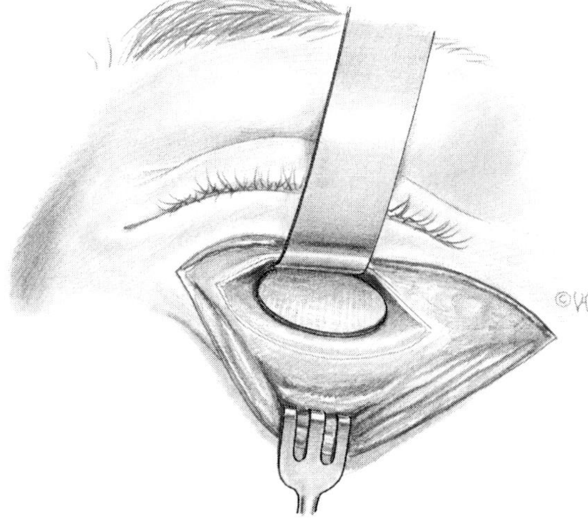

F, Orbital implant covering fracture site.

As a result of a force delivered to the bridge of the nose, the nasal bones are shattered, as well as the frontal process of the maxilla. As the impact continues, the lacrimal and ethmoid bones are fractured and are displaced laterally. The distance between the medial canthi is increased, a condition called traumatic telecanthus (Plate 18-3, *A*). Patients with these types of fractures are easy to identify, because they have flattened nasal bridges and laterally displaced medial canthi. If these patients are not seen soon after injury, which is often the case, the bone fragments are then malunited. Along with the destruction of the bony structures, the enclosed components of the lacrimal system are also disrupted.

To repair this area, an open reduction of the fracture with the reconstitution of the lacrimal system via dacryocystorhinostomy is necessary. The canthal tendons are replaced with transnasal wires.

General anesthesia is preferred for this procedure, but nonetheless the area is infiltrated with topical anesthesia containing epinephrine. Nasal packing with gauze soaked in 4% cocaine is also preferred at the start of the procedure.

Repair is begun by making a vertical incision about 3 to 5 mm nasal to the medial canthus and dissecting down to the level of the periosteum of the fractured area. The incision is extended as necessary to expose the length of the involved area. The lacrimal sac is then located. The bone in the area is stripped of periosteum with a periosteal elevator, if possible, and the lacrimal sac is reflected medially. The sac is usually swollen with mucopurulent material.

A drill is then used to create an osteotomy and at the same time to contour the medial canthal area (Plate 18-3, *B*). The lacrimal sac should be given adequate protection during the drilling procedure. When the nasal mucosa has been reached, flaps are prepared in it and in the lacrimal sac, as has been described for a dacryocystorhinostomy. The posterior flaps are sutured with 5-0 chromic catgut suture (Plate 18-3, *C*).

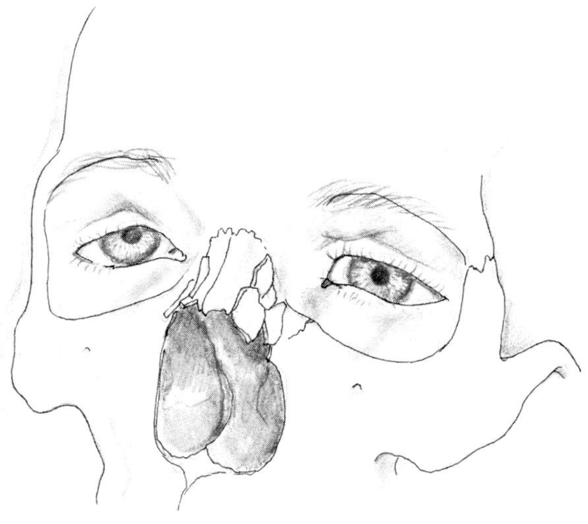

A, Bone displacement in naso-orbital fracture.

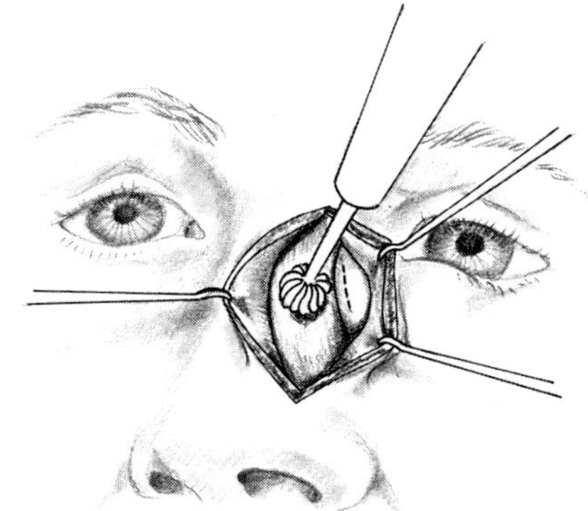

B, Burr used to create osteotomy.

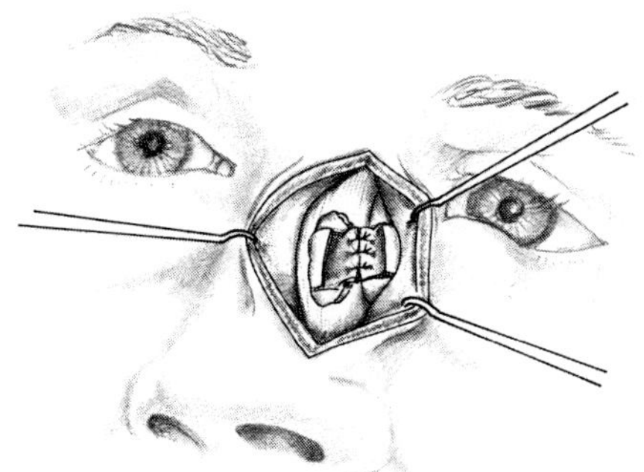

C, Posterior flaps created and sutured between lacrimal sac and lining of nasal bone.

At this point, the procedure is repeated on the contralateral side, which is usually involved in these fractures. The anterior flaps are sutured with absorbable suture. Next, an air drill is used to drill two holes through the bridge of the nose, one in line with the anterior lacrimal crest and one somewhat posterior, to realign the facial contour (Plate 18-3, *D*). Stainless steel wires are passed through the two holes and inserted through the medial canthal tendons on each side. The wires are tightened down to the nasal bridge by twisting them with a hemostat. They are cut with an appropriate wire cutter. The medial canthal tendons have now been repositioned (Plate 18-3, *E*). Two additional wires are now passed through the holes to emerge through the edges of the skin incision, one anterior and one posterior.

Subcutaneous layers are closed with 5-0 Vicryl sutures and the skin with interrupted 6-0 mild chromic sutures. The wire is then threaded through plastic plates and twisted to hold the plates in position against the medial canthus. These plates hold the underlying structures in position and relieve wound tension (Plate 18-3, *F*).

Light dressings are applied and then removed after 24 hours. Cold compresses are applied. The plastic plates are removed after a 2-week period.

Occasionally, nasal reconstruction is required with bone grafts from the iliac crest or ribs. We generally leave this work to a facial plastic surgeon or an ear, nose, and throat surgeon.

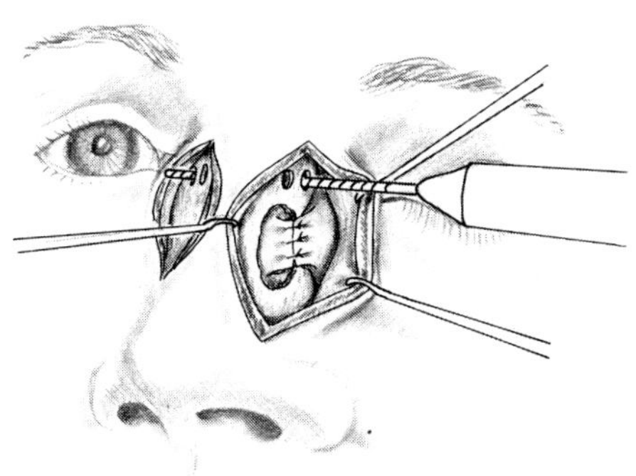

D, Anterior flaps sutured and holes drilled through bridge of nose.

E, Medial canthal tendons wired into position.

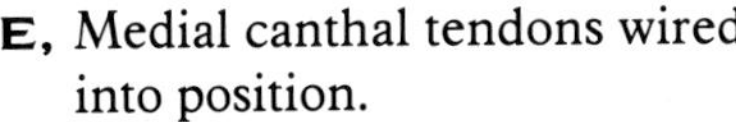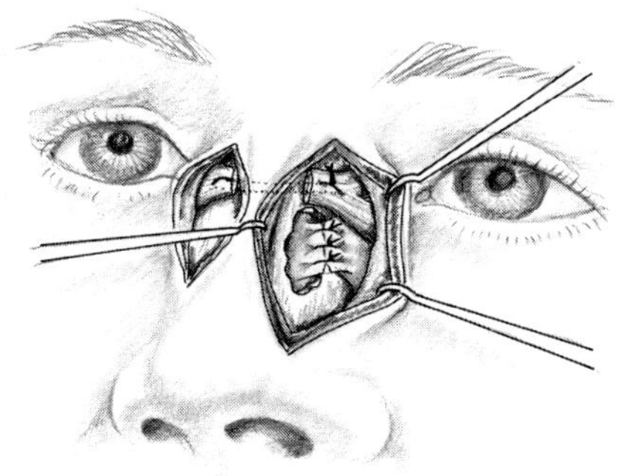

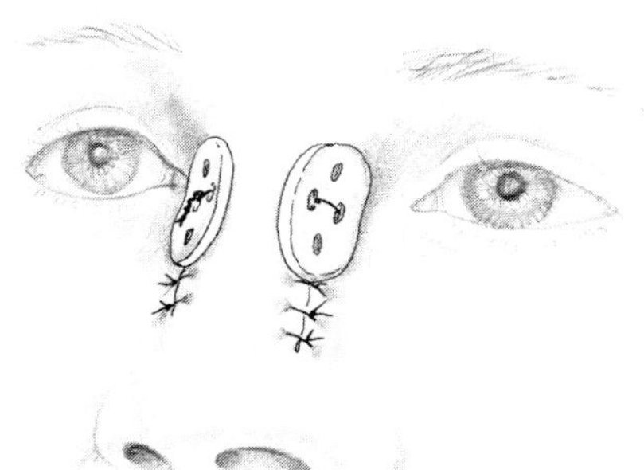

F, Plastic buttons wired into position and incisions closed.

ORBITAL TUMORS

Newer diagnostic techniques have greatly refined the preoperative evaluation of orbital masses. The use of orbital ultrasound and CT scans has made exploration and biopsy necessary in far fewer instances than before. However, it is still often necessary to seek tissue diagnoses to plan further treatment modalities. The diagnosis of a benign lesion may make partial excision or nonsurgical treatment a possibility, whereas a biopsy that suggests a growing mass indicates that more radical treatment is necessary.

Although masses that can be palpated through the lid are usually approachable through a transcutaneous incision, these tumors often extend deeply into the orbit. When these lesions are adherent to the globe or rectus muscles or both, the usual anterior orbital approaches (subciliary, superotemporal, superonasal, and lacrimal) may not offer adequate exposure and accessibility to the tumor. The approach that we prefer for handling tumors of this type is the transmarginal approach, in which the full thickness of the lid is incised to the fornix, affording complete accessibility to the mass (Plate 19-1, *A*). A palpable mass occupying the nasal one third of the upper lid may extend behind the medial canthal tendon (Plate 19-1, *B*) along the globe and medial rectus muscle (Plate 19-1, *C*).

In this procedure we normally prefer general anesthesia, although adequate local anesthesia can be achieved by using 2% lidocaine with 1:100,000 epinephrine.

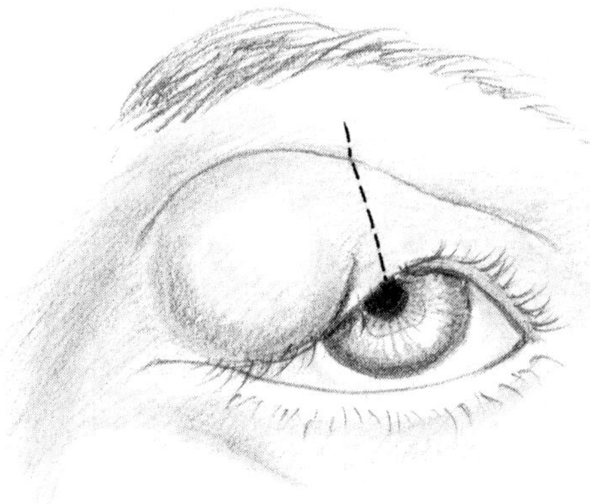

A, Anterior orbital tumor with area of transmarginal incision outlined.

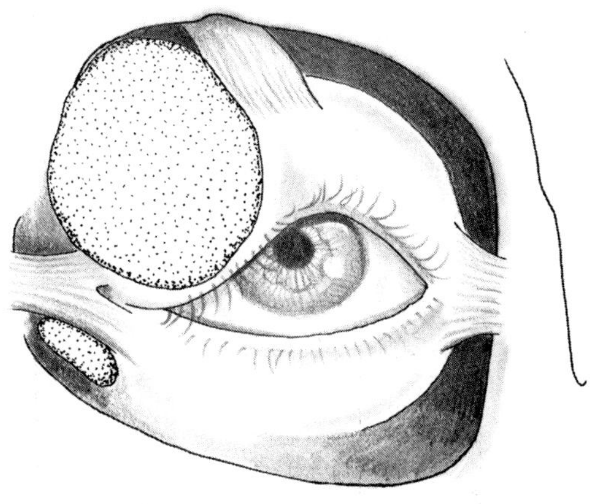

B, Intraorbital extent of tumor.

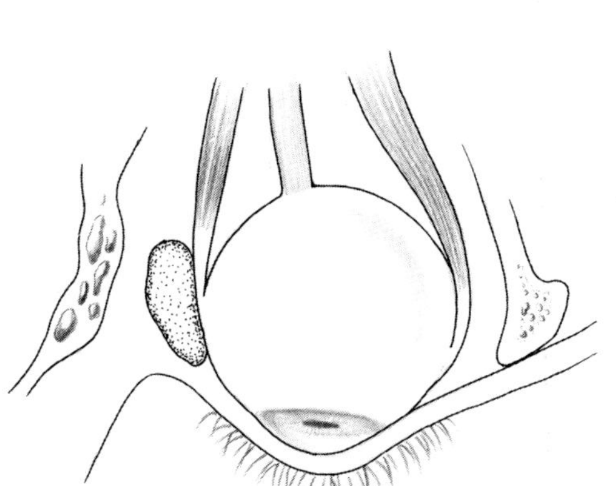

C, Relationship of tumor to medial rectus muscle.

With adequate protection for the globe, a full-thickness, vertical transmarginal incision is made with a no. 11 Bard-Parker blade down to the fornix in the area overlying the mass. To facilitate this incision, both sides of the area outlined for incision are grasped with forceps, and traction is exerted in a downward and outward direction. When the incision has reached the upper fornix, the lid flaps are turned outward and retracted with 4-0 silk sutures passed through the lid margins (Plate 19-1, *D*).

The anterior extent of the tumor is then visible. An incision is made through the conjunctiva from the superior apex of the lid incision, over the tumor mass and into the lower cul-de-sac. Care must be taken not to transversely incise and damage the levator aponeurosis or Müller's muscle in dissecting the tumor.

The mass is grasped with forceps and, while being gently retracted, is bluntly dissected from the underlying sclera and medial rectus muscle (Plate 19-1, *E*). After the mass has been carefully excised and adequate hemostasis achieved, the conjunctival layer is closed with continuous 8-0 Vicryl sutures (Plate 19-1, *F*). The full-thickness lid incision is closed with the three-suture technique (Plate 19-1, *G*). A light Telfa dressing is applied.

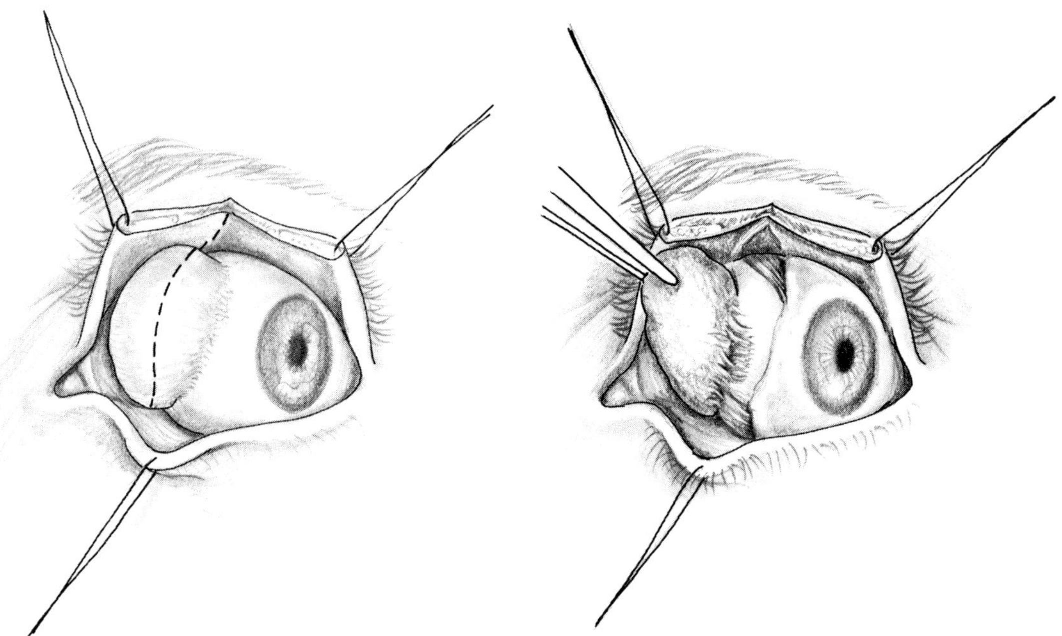

D, Following lid incision, extent of tumor is evident.

E, Excision of tumor from underlying tissue.

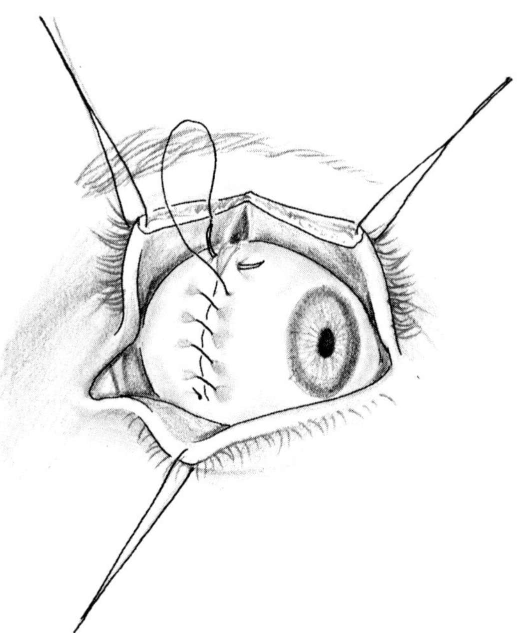

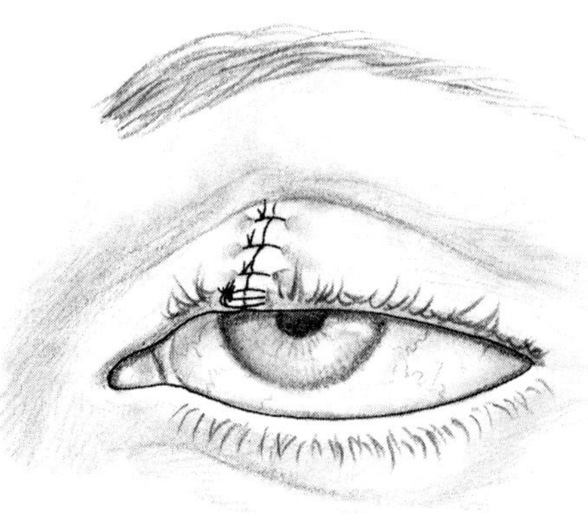

G, Transmarginal laceration closed.

F, Conjunctival layer of incision being closed.

The most useful procedure for exploration of the retrobulbar space is the lateral orbitotomy. This approach offers accessibility to tumors in the area between the periorbita and the muscle cone and within the muscle cone. In addition, the lateral orbitotomy is the procedure of choice for excision of tumors that are located posteriorly and anterior tumors with posterior extension.

This procedure is performed with the patient under general anesthesia. Appropriate antibiotics are infused preoperatively. The lateral eyelids and brow are infiltrated with 1% lidocaine with 1:100,000 epinephrine. An S-shaped incision with a no. 15 Bard-Parker blade is begun just beneath the lateral half of the eyebrow and extended infero-laterally along the outer edge of the lateral orbital rim. It turns posteriorly just past the lateral canthal angle (Plate 19-2, *A*). The lateral orbital rim is identified. The skin and subcutaneous tissues are undermined above and below the incision. The wound edges are retracted, usually with a self-retaining retractor.

At this point, a 6-0 silk suture is passed through the lateral rectus muscle, and the globe is rotated medially. Malleable retractors are used to expose the muscle layer (Plate 19-2, *B*). At the periosteal level, a Bard-Parker blade is used to incise the periosteum, which is reflected from the bone (Plate 19-2, *C* and *D*). This incision is made parallel to the margin of the lateral orbital rim and is extended 10 mm above and below the horizontal canthal incision. A periosteal elevator is helpful in making the dissection.

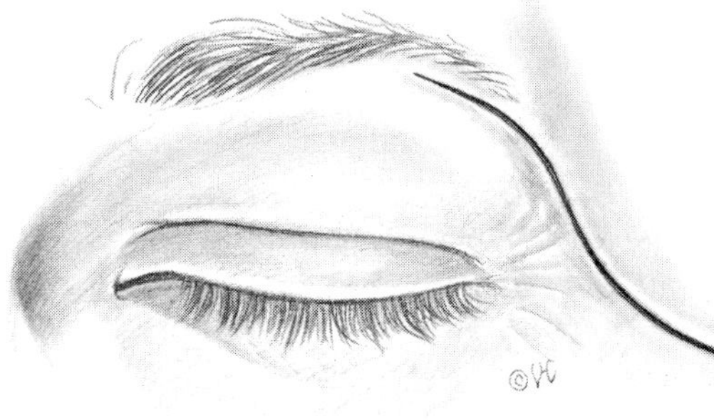

A, S-shaped incision made to expose lateral orbital rim.

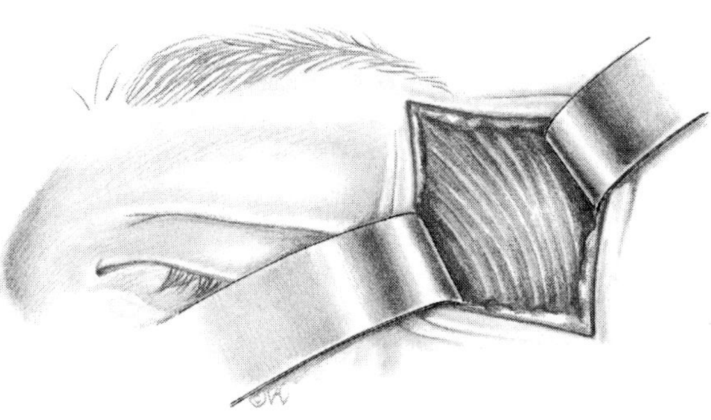

B, Retractors used to expose muscle layer.

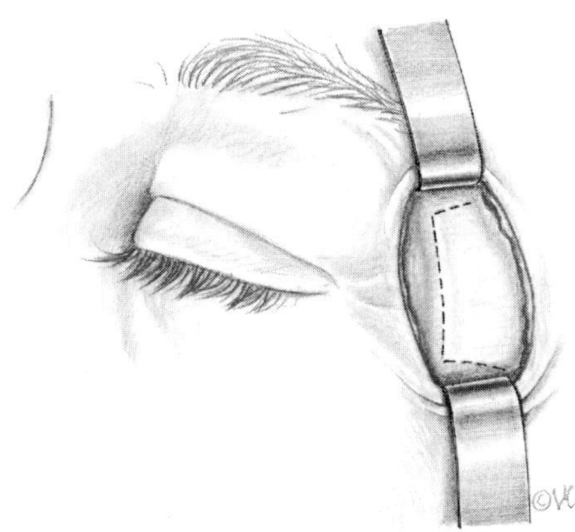

C, Periosteum to be incised.

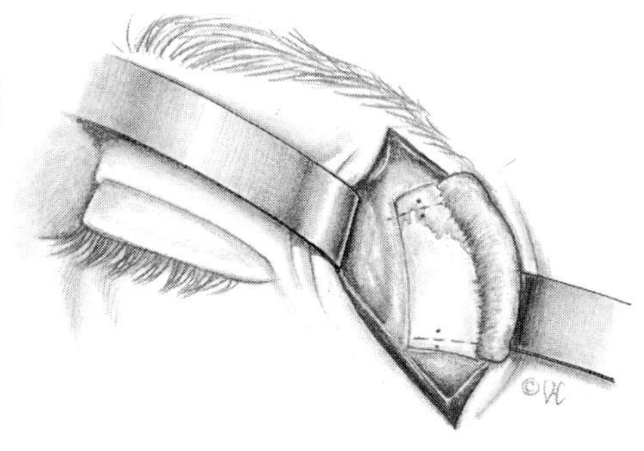

D, Periosteum incised and reflected temporally.

A bone flap about 20 mm long is then created on the lateral orbital wall and mobilized.

A Stryker saw is used to cut through the lateral orbital rim. The globe should be adequately protected at this time with a ribbon retractor or lid plate. The Stryker saw should be angled so that the superior cut is turned downward to avoid the cranial vault. The lower cut is angled slightly upward so that the saw enters the orbit and not the maxillary bone (Plate 19-2, *E*).

The lateral orbital rim is then grasped and reflected posteriorly, with the thin bone of the temporal fossa cracking easily (Plate 19-2, *F*). This bone flap may be removed or rotated outward. We prefer to remove the bone, because this permits some expansion of the orbital contents postoperatively. This approach also gives good exposure and access to the retroorbital space. If necessary, the bony opening can be increased in size with a rongeur.

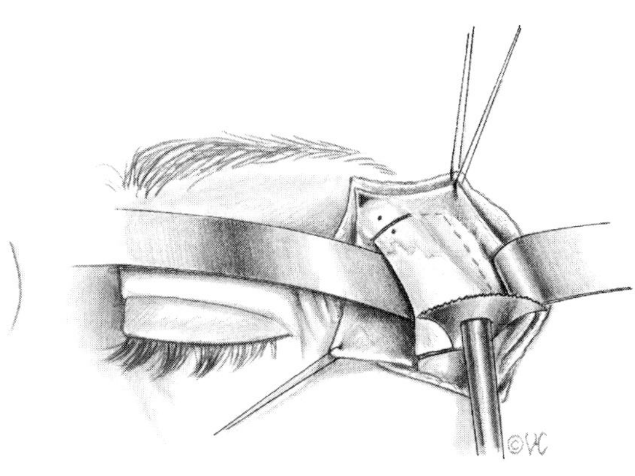

E, Stryker saw used to create bone flap while plate protects globe.

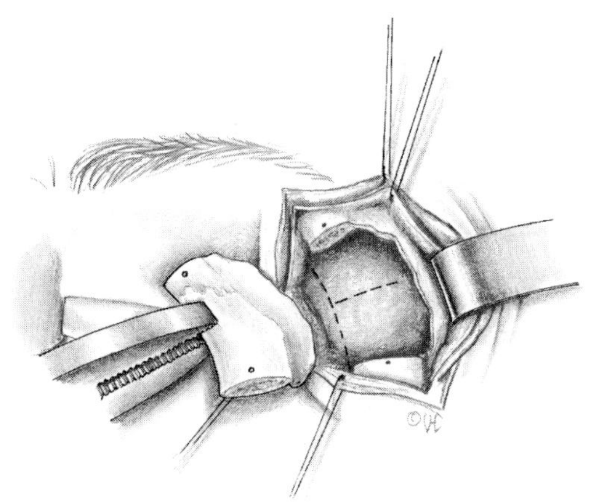

F, Bone flap is removed.

The periorbita is now visible. It is carefully cut and separated with a horizontal incision (Plate 19-2, *G* and *H*). Exploration of the orbit should be performed with the utmost care. Even encapsulated masses should be so handled. A cryoprobe is often used. Hemostasis should be meticulously maintained at all times. The lateral rectus muscle is usually located at this time and a suture passed around it so that it can be retracted (Plate 19-2, *I*). The operative site is carefully packed (Plate 19-2, *J*).

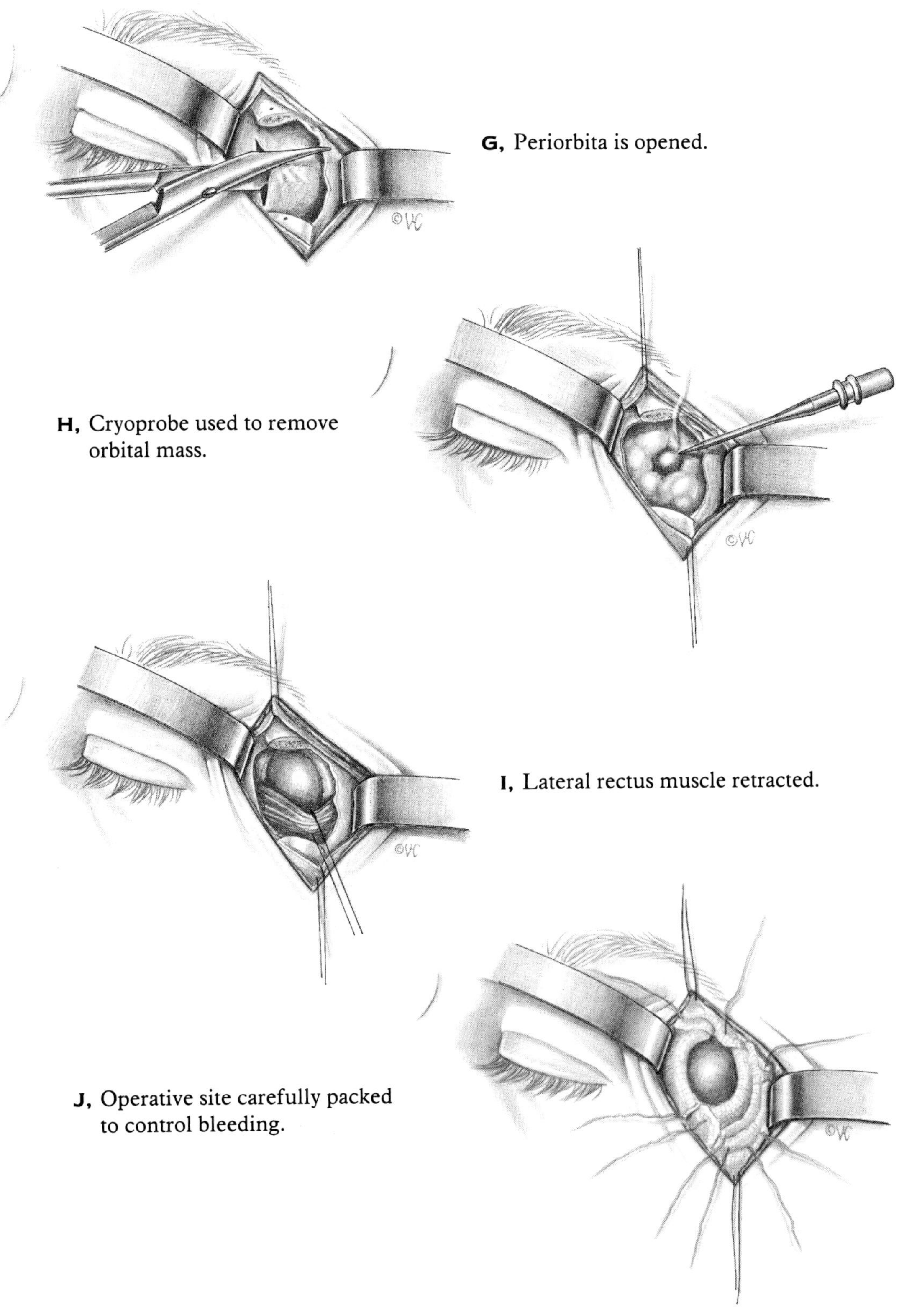

G, Periorbita is opened.

H, Cryoprobe used to remove orbital mass.

I, Lateral rectus muscle retracted.

J, Operative site carefully packed to control bleeding.

If the bone flap is replaced, it should be secured with 4-0 Mesilene sutures (Plate 19-2, *K*). The suture holes are easiest to drill before the bone is removed from its original position (Plate 19-2, *L* and *M*). Interrupted 5-0 Vicryl sutures are used to close the subcutaneous tissues (Plate 19-2, *N*). A small drain may be placed into the orbit before the skin is closed (Plate 18-2, *N*. It may be advanced slowly, according to the volume of drainage. It can usually be removed after 1 or 2 days. The skin is closed with running, intradermal 6-0 nylon sutures. A pressure bandage may be placed laterally, but not over the eye. The vision should be checked every 15 minutes postoperatively for 2 to 3 hours. It should be counting fingers or better unless the preoperative vision was worse.

The wound is closed with 5-0 chromic catgut suture used for the subcutaneous tissue. If the bone flap is replaced, it need not be wired. The skin is closed with 6-0 silk suture. A light dressing is applied.

Postoperatively the dressing is changed daily for several days. The silk sutures are removed after 4 to 5 days.

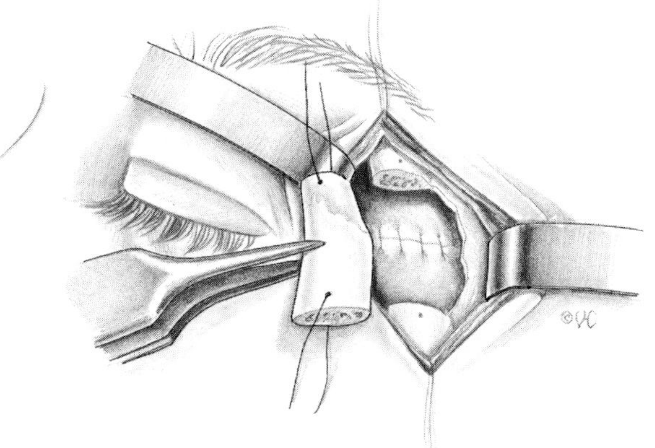

K, Bone flap can be replaced.

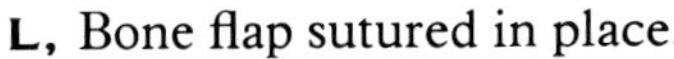

L, Bone flap sutured in place.

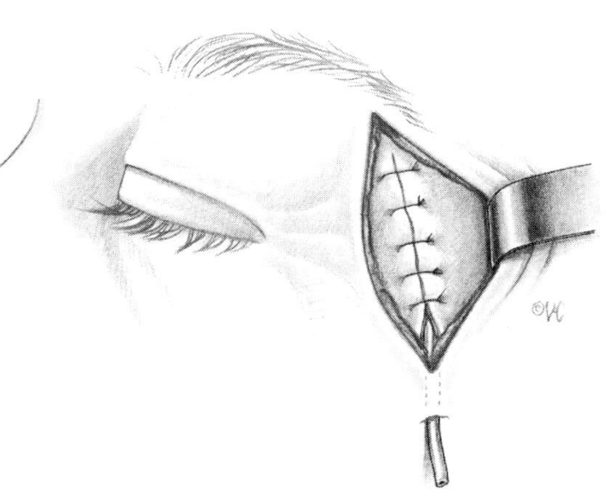

M, Subcutaneous tissue closed and small drain inserted.

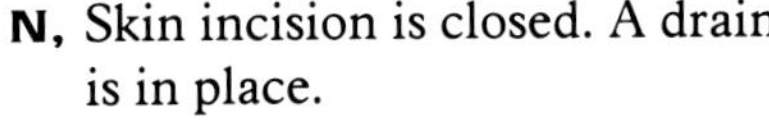

N, Skin incision is closed. A drain is in place.

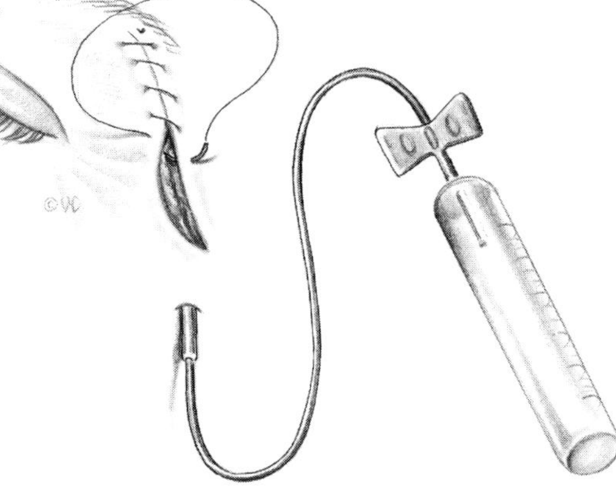

BIBLIOGRAPHY

CHAPTER 2

1. Anderson RL: Medial canthal tendon branches out, Arch Ophthalmol 95:2051, 1977.
2. Anderson RL, Dixon RS: The role of Whitnall's ligament in ptosis surgery, Arch Ophthalmol 97:705, 1979.
3. Bailey JH: Surgical anatomy of the lacrimal sac, Am J Ophthalmol 6:665, 1923.
4. Bergen MR: Relationship between the arteries and veins and the connective tissue system in the human orbit, parts I, II, III, Acta Morphol Neerl Scand 28:1, 1982.
5. Corin SM, Hurwitz JJ, Jaffer N, Botta EP: The true canalicular angle: a mathematical model, Ophthalmic Plast Reconstr Surg 6:42-45, 1990.
6. Hargiss JJ: Surgical anatomy of the eyelids, Trans Pacif Coast Otolaryngol Soc 44:193, 1963.
7. Hawes MJ, Dortzbach RK: The microscopic anatomy of the lower eyelid retractors, Arch Ophthalmol 100:1313, 1982.
8. Horner WE: Description of a small muscle at the internal commissure of the eyelids, Philadelphia J Med Phys Sci 8:70, 1824.
9. Jones JT: An anatomical approach to problems of the eyelids and lacrimal apparatus, Arch Ophthalmol 66:111, 1961.
10. Lockwood CB: The anatomy of the muscles, ligaments, and fascia of the orbit, including an account of the capsule of tenon, the check ligaments of recti, and of the suspensory ligament of the eye, J Anat Physiol 20:1, 1886.
11. Meyer DR, Linberg JV, Wobig JL, McCormick SA: Anatomy of the orbital septum and associated eyelid connective tissues: implications for ptosis surgery, Ophthalmic Plast Surg 7:104-113, 1991.
12. Thaller SR, Kim S, Patterson H, Wildman M, Daniller A: The submuscular aponeurotic system (SMAS): a histologic and comparative anatomy evaluation, Plast Reconstr Surg 86:690-695, 1990.
13. Warwick R: Eugene Wolff's anatomy of the eyelids and orbit, ed 7, Philadelphia, 1976, WB Saunders.
14. Whitnall SE, Anatomy of the human orbit, London, 1932, Oxford University Press.
15. Williams, PL, Warwick R, editors: Gray's anatomy, ed 36, Philadelphia, 1980, WB Saunders.

CHAPTER 3

1. Artz JS, Dinner MI, Foglietti MA: Planning the aesthetic foreheadplasty, Ann Plast Surg 25:1-6, 1990.
2. Borges AF, Alexander JE: Relaxed skin tension lines, Z-plasties on scars, and fusiform excision of lesions, Br J Plast Surg 15:242, 1962.
3. Borges AF, Gibson T: The original Z-plasty, Br J Plast Surg 16:379, 1963.
4. Converse JM, editor: Reconstructive Plastic Surgery ed 2, vol 1, Philadelphia, 1977, WB Saunders.
5. McCord CD, Doxanas MT: Browplasty and browpexy: an adjunct to blepharoplasty, Plast Reconstr Surg 86:248-254, 1990.
6. McGregor IA: Fundamental techniques of plastic surgery, ed 6, Edinburgh, 1975, Churchill Livingstone.
7. Middleton DG, McCullach C: An enquiry into characteristics of sutures, particularly fine sutures, Advan Ophthalmol 22:35, 1970.
8. Mathog RH: Basic management of soft tissue injury. In Spoor TC, Nesi FA, editors: Management of ocular, orbital, and adnexal trauma, New York, 1988, Raven Press, pp 365-379.
9. Wyngaarden JB, Smith LH: Cecil texbtook of medicine, ed 16, Philadelphia, 1982, WB Saunders.

CHAPTER 4

1. Converse JM: Introduction to plastic surgery. In Converse JM, editor: Reconstructive plastic surgery, vol 2, Philadelphia, 1964, WB Saunders.

2. Garber PF: Lateral canthoplasty. In Smith B, Bosniak S, editors: Advances in ophthalmic plastic surgery, vol 2, Elmsford NJ, 1983, Pergamon Press.

3. Hurwitz JJ, Archer KF, Gruss JS: Treatment of severe lower eyelid retraction with scleral and free skin grafts and bipedicle orbicularis flap, Ophthalmic Surg 21:167-172, 1990.

4. Loeffler M, Hornblass A: Surgical management of congenital upper eyelid eversion, Ophthalmic Surg 21:435-437, 1990.

CHAPTER 5

1. Beyer CK: Lid and canalicular trauma. In Freeman HM, editor: Ocular trauma, New York, 1979, Appleton-Century-Crofts.

2. Crawford J: Intubation of the lacrimal system, Ophthalmic Plast Reconstr Surg 5:261-265, 1989.

3. Daubert J, Nik N, Chandeyssoun P, El-Choufi L: Tear flow analysis through the upper and lower systems, Ophthalmic Plast Reconstr Surg 6:193-196, 1990.

4. Dibble RF, Friedel SD: A simplified method of monocanalicular silicone intubation, Ophthalmic Surg 21:134-135, 1990.

5. Eccarius SG, Gordon MF, Parelman JJ: Bicarbonate-buffered lidocaine-epinephrine-hyaluronidase for eyelid anesthesia, Ophthalmology 97:1499-1501, 1990.

6. Flanagan JC: Trauma: eyelid complications, Trans Pa Acad Ophthalmol Otolaryngol 33:156, 1980.

7. Goldberg MF, Tessler HH: Occult intraocular perforations from brow and lid lacerations, Arch Ophthalmol 86:145, 1971.

8. Jones NP: Perforating eye injuries caused by dog bites, J R Soc Med 83:332-333, 1990.

9. Ramocki JR, Nesi FA, Spoor TC: Management of injuries to the ocular adnexa. In Spoor TC, Nesi FA, editors: Management of ocular, orbital, and adnexal trauma, New York, 1988, Raven Press, pp 381-426.

10. Saunders PH, Shannon CM, Flanagan JC: The effectiveness of pigtail probe method of repairing canalicular lacerations, Ophthalmic Surg 9:33, 1978.

11. Serrano F, Stack T, Esquenazi S: Surgical treatment of human bites of the upper eyelid, Ophthalmic Plast Reconstr Surg 5:127-130, 1989.

12. Smith BC, Nesi FA: Upper eyelid loss due to formalin injection: surgical reconstruction, Trans Am Acad Ophthalmol Otolaryngol 86:1951, 1979.

CHAPTER 6

1. Chalfin J, Putterman AM: Frozen section control in the surgery of basal cell carcinoma of the eyelid, Am J Ophthalmol 87:802, 1979.

2. Clark WH Jr et al: The histogenesis and biologic behavior of primary human malignant melanoma of the skin, Cancer Res 29:705, 1969.

3. Doxanas MT, Green WR, Iliff CE: Factors in the successful management of basal cell carcinomas of the eyelids, Am J Ophthalmol 91:726, 1981.

4. Gunnarson G, Larko O, Hersle K: Cryosurgery of eyelid basal cell carcinomas, Acta Ophthalmol 68:241-245, 1990.

5. Henkind P, Friedman A: Cancer of the lids and ocular adnexa. In Andrade R et al, editors: Cancer of the skin, Philadelphia, 1926, WB Saunders.

6. Jakobiec FA, Iwamoto T: The ocular adnexa: lids, conjunctiva, and orbit. In Fine B, Yanoff M, editors: Histology: a text and atlas, Hagarstown, Md, 1978, Harper & Row.

7. Kopf AW et al: Curettage-electrodessication treatment of basal cell carcinoma, Arch Dermatol 113:439, 1977.

8. Korn E: Use of a carbon dioxide laser for lesions extending into the lashes, Ophthalmic Surg 21:581-584, 1990.

9. Leibsohn J, Bullock J, Waller R: Full thickness eyelid biopsy for presumed carcinoma in situ of the palpebral conjunctiva, Ophthalmol Surg 13:840, 1982.

10. Shields JA: Secondary orbital tumors. In Diagnosis and management of orbital tumors, Philadelpha, 1989, WB Saunders, pp 341-377.

CHAPTER 7

1. Anderson RL, Edwards JJ: Reconstruction by myocutaneous eyelid flaps, Arch Ophthalmol 97:2358, 1979.

2. Becker FF: Surgery of the medial canthal region, Ann Plast Surg 7:258, 1981.

3. Callahan MA, Callahan A: Ophthalmic Plastic and Orbital Surgery, Birmingham, Ala, 1979, Aesculpius.

4. Chiarelli A, Baldelli A, Di Vincenzo A: Utilization of the superficial temporoparietal fascia in reconstructive plastic surgery: a clinical case, Ophthalmic Plast Reconstr Surg 5:274-276, 1989.

5. Cutler NL, Beard C: A method for partial and total upper lid reconstruction, Am J Ophthalmol 39:1, 1955.

6. Hughes WL: Reconstruction of the lid, Am J Ophthalmol 28:1203, 1945.
7. Leone CR: Nasal septal cartilage for eyelid reconstruction, Ophthalmic Surg 4:68, 1973.
8. Leone CR: Tarsal conjunctival advancement flaps for upper eyelid reconstruction, Arch Ophthalmol 101:945, 1983.
9. McCord CD, Nunery WR: Reconstructive procedures of the lower eyelid and outer canthus. In McCord CD Jr, editor: Oculoplastic Surgery, ed 2, New York, 1987, Raven Press, pp 189-209.
10. McCord CD, Wesley RE: Reconstruction of the upper eyelid and medial canthus. In McCord CD Jr, editor: Oculoplastic Surgery, ed 2, New York, 1987, Raven Press, pp 175-188.
11. Mustardé JC: Eyelid reconstruction, Orbit 1:33, 1982.
12. Patrinely JR, Marines HM, Anderson RL: Skin flaps in periorbital reconstruction, Surv Ophthalmol 31:249-261, 1987.
13. Small RG, Sahl WJ: The use of split-thickness skin grafts for eyelid reconstruction after Mohs' fresh-tissue surgery, Ophthalmic Plast Reconstr Surg 5:266-270, 1989.
14. Smith B: Eyelid surgery, Surg Clin North Am 39:77, 1959.
15. Smith B, Beyer CK: Medial canthoplasty, Arch Ophthalmol 82:344, 1969.
16. Smith B, Lisman RD: Auricular cartilage grafts, split thickness, Ophthalmic Surg 13:1018, 1982.
17. Tijl JWM, Koorneef L: Optimal follow-up time for a basal cell carcinoma of the eyelid, Doc Ophthalmol 75:275-279, 1990.
18. Tenzel RR, Stewart WB: Eyelid reconstruction by semicircular flap technique, Trans Am Soc Ophthalmol Otolaryngol 85:1165, 1978.
19. Wesley RE, McCord CD: Transplantation of eyebank sclera in the Cutler-Beard method of upper eyelid reconstruction, Ophthalmology 87:1022, 1980.

CHAPTER 8

1. Collins JR, Rathbun JE: Involutional entropion: a review with evaluation of a procedure, Arch Ophthalmol 96:1056, 1978.
2. Dortzbach RK, McGetrick JJ: Involutional entropion of the lower eyelid, Adv Ophth Plast Reconstr Surg 2:257, 1985.
3. Hurwitz JJ, Smith D, Corwin SM: Association of entropion with cataract surgery, Ophthalmic Plast Reconstr Surg 6:25-27, 1990.
4. McCord CD, Chen WP: Tarsal polishing and mucous membrane grafting for cicatricial entropion, trichiasis, and epidermalization, Ophthalmic Surg 14:1021, 1983.
5. Miller DG, Hesse RJ: Involutional entropion of the upper lid, Ophthalmic Plast Reconstr Surg 6:16-20, 1990.
6. Rosenberg S, Sanchez M: Mideyelid entropion, Ophthalmic Plast Reconst Surg 6:21-24, 1990.
7. Wagemans MJ, Koorneef L: A new and simple approach to the treatment of both entropion and ectropion: the double pentagonal wedge, Orbit 8:249-252, 1989.
8. Wies FA: Spastic entropion, Trans Am Acad Ophthalmol Otolaryngol 59:503, 1955.

CHAPTER 9

1. Anderson RL, Gordy DD: The tarsal strip procedure, Arch Ophthalmol 97:2192, 1979.
2. Converse JM: Introduction to plastic surgery. In Converse JM, editor: Reconstructive plastic surgery, vol 2, Philadelphia, 1964, WB Saunders.
3. Edelstein JP, Dryden RM: Medial palpebral tendon repair for medial ectropion of the lower eyelid, Ophthalmic Plast Reconstr Surg 6:28-37, 1990.
4. Hurwitz JJ, Archer KF, Gruss JS: Treatment of severe lower eyelid retraction with scleral and free skin grafts and bipedicle orbicularis flap, Ophthalmic Surg 21:167-172, 1990.
5. Hurwitz JJ, Tucker S: Posterior horizontal and vertical tightening to treat combined punctal ectropion with medial canthal tendon laxity, Ophthalmic Surg 21:721-725, 1990.
6. Levin ML, Leone CR Jr: Bipedicle myocutaneous flap repair of cicatricial ectropion, Ophthalmic Plast Reconstr Surg 6:119-121, 1990.
7. Sisler HA, Lebay GR, Finlay JR: Senile ectropion and entropion: a comparative histopathologic study, Ann Ophthalmol 8:319, 1976.
8. Smith B: The "Lazy-T" correction of ectropion of the lower punctum, Arch Ophthalmol 94:1149, 1976.
9. Tse D: Surgical correction of punctal malposition, Am J Ophthalmol 100:339, 1985.

CHAPTER 10

1. Baker TJ, Gordon HL, Mosienko P: Upper lid blepharoplasty, Plast Reconstr Surg 60:692, 1977.
2. Beekhuis GJ: Blepharoplasty, Otolaryngol Clin North Am 131:225, 1980.
3. Beyer CK, McCarthy RW, Webster RC: Baggy lids: a classification and newer aspects of treatment to avoid complications, Ophthalmic Surg 11:169, 1980.

4. Goldberg RA, Marmor MF, Shorr N, Christenbury JD: Blindness following blepharoplasty: two case reports, and a discussion of management, Ophthalmic Surg 21:85-89, 1990.
5. Jones LT, Wobig JL: Surgery of the eyelids and lacrimal system, Birmingham Ala, 1976, Aesculapius.
6. Jordan DR: The blepharochalasis syndrome, Arch Ophthalmol 108:1633, 1990.
7. Mandel MA: Closure of blepharoplasty incisions with autologous fibrin glue, Arch Ophthalmol 108:842-844, 1990.
8. Massima H: Combined skin and skin-muscle flap technique in lower blepharoplasty: a 10-year experience, Ann Plast Surg 25:467-476, 1990.
9. May JW, Fearon J, Zingarelli P: Retro-orbicularis oculus fat (ROOF) resection in aesthetic blepharoplasty: a 6-year study in 63 patients, Plast Reconstr Surg 86:682-689, 1990.
10. McCord CD, Doxanas MT: Browplasty and browpexy: an adjunct to blepharoplasty, Plast Reconstr Surg 86:248-254, 1990.
11. Neuhaus RW, Baylis HJ: Complications of lower eyelid blepharoplasty. In Putterman AM, editor: Cosmetic oculoplastic surgery, New York, 1982, Grune & Stratton.
12. Putterman AM: Patient satisfaction in oculoplastic surgery, Ophthalmic Surgery 21:15-21, 1990.
13. Putterman AM, Urist MJ: Baggy eyelids: a true hernia, Ann Ophthalmol 5:1029, 1973.
14. Sheen JH: Tarsal fixation in lower blepharoplasty, Plast Reconstr Surg 62:64, 1981.
15. Small RG: Extended lower eyelid blepharoplasty, Arch Ophthalmol 99:1042, 1981.
16. Smith B, Bosniak SL: Reconstructing the supratarsal crease, Adv Ophthalmol Plast Reconstr Surg 1:75, 1982.
17. Tenzel R: Complications of cosmetic blepharoplasty. In Smith BC, Guibor P: Contemporary Oculopastic Surgery New York, 1974, Stratton Intercontinental Medical Book Corp.
18. Webster RC, Davidson TM, Smith RC: Wound closure with absorbable sutures, Laryngoscope 86:1280, 1976.

CHAPTER 12

1. Arden R, Mathog R, Nesi F: Flap reconstruction techniques in conjunctivorhinostomy, Otolaryngol Head Neck Surg 102:150-155, 1990.
2. Bartley G, Gustafson R: Complications of malpositioned Jones tubes, Am J Ophthalmol 109:66-69, 1990.
3. Carroll JM, Beyer C: Conjunctivodacryocystorhinostomy using silicone rubber lacrimal tubes, Arch Ophthalmol 89:113, 1973.
4. Crawford J: Intubation of the lacrimal system, Ophthalmic Plast Reconstr Surg 5:261-265, 1989.
5. Daubert J, Nik N, Chandeyssoun P, El-Chouri L: Tear flow analysis through the upper and lower systems, Ophthalmic Plast Reconstr Surg 6:193-196, 1990.
6. Dibble RF, Friedel SD: A simplified method of monocanalicular silicone intubation, Ophthalmic Surg 21:134-135, 1990.
7. Gonnering R, Lyon D, Fisher J: Endoscopic laser-assisted lacrimal surgery, Am J Ophthalmol 111:152-157, 1991.
8. Jones LT: An anatomic approach to problems of the eyelids and lacrimal apparatus, Arch Opthalmol 66:111, 1961.
9. Leone C, Van Gemert J: The success rate of silicone intubation in congenital lacrimal obstruction, Ophthalmic Surg 21:90-92, 1990.
10. Manrube del Castillo J: Conjunctivorhinostomy without osteal perforation, Arch Ophthalmol 100:310, 1982.
11. Nixon J, Birchall IWJ, Virjee J: The role of dacryocystography in the management of patients with epiphora, Br J Radiol 63:337-339, 1990.
12. Orcutt J, Hillel A, Weymuller E: Endoscopic repair of failed dacryocystorhinostomy, Ophthalmic Plast Reconstr Surg 6:197-202, 1990.
13. Welsh M, Katowitz J: Timing of Silastic tubing removal after intubation for congenital nasolacrimal duct obstruction, Ophthalmic Plast Reconstr Surg 5:43-48, 1990.

CHAPTER 13

1. Anderson RL: Age of aponeurotic awareness, Ophthalmic Plast Reconstr Surg 1:77, 1985.
2. Anderson RL, Dixon RS: Aponeurotic ptosis surgery, Arch Ophthalmol 97:1123, 1979.
3. Anderson RL, Jordan DR, Dutton JJ: Whitnall's sling for poor function ptosis, Arch Ophthalmol 108:1628-1632, 1990.
4. Beard C: Ptosis, St Louis, 1980, Mosby–Year Book.
5. Berke RN, Wadsworth JAC: Histology of levator muscle in congenital and acquired ptosis, Arch Ophthalmol 53:413, 1955.

6. Crawford JS: Repair of ptosis using frontalis muscle and fascia lata, Trans Am Acad Ophthalmol Otolaryngol 60:627, 1956.

7. De Blaskovics L: A new operation for ptosis with shortening of the levator tarsus, Arch Ophthalmol 52:563, 1923.

8. Dortzbach RK, McGetrick JJ: Diagnosis and treatment of acquired ptosis, Module 10, Focal Points 1984, American Academy of Ophthalmology.

9. Dortzbach RK, Sutula FC: Involutional blepharoptosis: a histopathologic study, Arch Ophthalmol 98:2045, 1980.

10. Downes RN, Collin JRO: The Mersilene mesh ptosis sling, Eye 4:456-463, 1990.

11. Eccarius SG, Gordon ME, Parelman JJ: Bicarbonate-buffered lidocaine-epinephrine-hyaluronidase for eyelid anesthesia, Ophthalmology 97:1449-1501, 1990.

12. Freuh BR: The mechanistic classification of ptosis, Ophthalmology 87:1019, 1980.

13. Galvaris PG: Minimal ptosis surgery. In Bosniak SL, Smith BC, editors: Advances in ophthalmic plastic and reconstructive surgery, vol 1, New York, 1982, Pergammon Press.

14. Jones LT, Quickert MH, Wobig JL: The cure of ptosis by aponeurotic repair, Arch Ophthalmol 93:629, 1975.

15. Jordan DT, Anderson RL: The aponeurotic approach to congenital ptosis, Ophthalmic Surg 21:237-244, 1990.

16. Levine MR: Short fascial strip—what next? Arch Ophthalmol 95:1621, 1977.

17. Mustardé JC: Problems and possibilities in ptosis surgery, Plast Reconstr Surg 56:381, 1975.

18. Putterman AM, Trist MJ: Mueller's muscle-conjunctiva resection, Arch Ophthalmol 93:629, 1975.

19. Servat J et al: The Fasanella-Servat operation: 1961-1981. In Bosniak SG, Smith BC, editors: Advances in ophthalmic plastic and reconstructive surgery, vol 1, New York, 1982, Pergamon Press.

20. Spoor TC, Quitko GM: Blepharoptosis repair by fascia lata suspension with direct tarsal and frontalis fixation, Am J Ophthalmol 109:314-317, 1990.

CHAPTER 14

1. Arion HG: Dynamic closure of the lids in paralysis of the orbicularis muscle, Int Surg 57:48, 1972.

2. Fernandez E, Pallini R, Maira G: Alternative to tarsorrhaphy in peripheral facial nerve palsy with expectation of functional recovery, J Neurosurg 61:405-406, 1984.

3. Fox SA: Temporary paracentral tarsorrhaphies. In Ophthalmic Plast Surgery New York, 1986, Grune & Stratton, pp 118-119.

4. Grove AS: Marginal tarsorrhaphy: a technique to minimize premature eyelid separation, Ophthalmic Surg 8:56-59, 1977.

5. Jelks GW, Smith B, Bosniak S: The evaluation and management of the eye in facial palsy, Clin Plast Surg 6:397-419, 1979.

6. Jobe RP: A technique for lid-loading in the management of lagophthalmos in facial paralysis, Plast Reconstr Surg 53:29-31, 1974.

7. Levine RE: Protection of the exposed eye. In Brackmann DE, editor: Neurological surgery of the ear and skull base, New York, 1982, Raven Press, pp 81-87.

8. Levine RE: Eyelid reanimation surgery. In May M, editor: The facial nerve, New York, 1986, Thieme-Stratton, pp 681-694.

9. May M: Surgical rehabilitation of facial palsy: total approach. In May M, editor: The facial nerve, New York, 1986, Thieme-Stratton, pp 695-777.

10. May M: Gold weight and wire spring implants as alternatives to tarsorrhaphy, Arch Otolaryngol Head Neck Surg 113:656-660, 1987.

11. Stamler JF, Tse DT: A simple and reliable technique for permanent lateral tarsorrhaphy, Arch Ophthalmol 108:125-127, 1990.

CHAPTER 15

1. Denig R: Transplantation of mucous membrane of the mouth for various diseases and burns of the cornea, NY State J Med 107:1074, 1918.

2. Fein W: Repair of total and subtotal symblepharon, Ophthalmic Surg 10:44, 1979.

3. Gould HL: Molded flush-fitting acrylic shells in ocular surgery. In Smith B, Converse JM, editors: Proceedings of the Second International Symposium on Plastic and Reconstructive Surgery of the Eye and Adnexa, St. Louis, 1967, Mosby—Year Book, pp 412-431.

4. Ralph RA: Reconstruction of conjunctival fornices using silicone rubber sheets, Ophthalmic Surg 6:55, 1975.

CHAPTER 16

1. Barraquer JI: Etiology, pathogenesis, and treatment of the pterygium. In Symposium on med-

ical and surgical diseases of the cornea: Transactions of the New Orleans Academy of Ophthalmology, St Louis, 1980, Mosby–Year Book, pp 167-178.
2. Fine M: Recurrent pterygium: mucous membrane grafts. In Symposium on medical and surgical diseases of the cornea: transactions of the New Orleans Academy of Ophthalmology, St Louis, 1980, Mosby–Year Book, pp 533-540.
3. Paton D: Pterygium management based upon a theory of pathogenesis, Trans Am Acad Ophthalmol Otolaryngol 79:603-612, 1975.
4. Pinkerton OD, Hokama Y, Shigemura LA: Immunologic basis for the pathogenesis of pterygium, Am J Ophthalmol 98:225-228, 1984.

CHAPTER 17

1. Bello VM, Levine MR: Superior sulcus deformity, Arch Ophthalmol 98:215-219, 1980.
2. Dutton JJ: Coraline hydroxyapatite as an ocular implant, Ophthalmology 98:370-377, 1991.
3. Kronish JW, Gonnering RS, Dortzbach RK, Rankin JHG, Reid DL, Phernetton TM: The pathophysiology of the anophthalmic socket: I. Analysis of orbital blood flow, Ophthalmic Plast Reconstr Surg 6:77-87, 1990.
4. Kronish JW et al: The pathophysiology of the anophthalmic socket. II. Analysis of orbital fat, Ophthalmic Plast Reconstr Surg 6:88-95, 1990.
5. McCord CD Jr, Moses JL: Exposure of the inferior orbit with fornix incision and lateral canthotomy, Ophthalmic Surg 10:53, 1979.
6. Perry AC: Integrated orbital implants, Adv Ophthalmic Plast Reconstr Surg 8:75-81, 1990.
7. Perry AC: Advances in enucleation, Ophthalmol Clin North Am 4:173-182, 1991.
8. Rose GE, Sigurdsson H, Collin R: The volume deficient orbit: clinical characteristics, surgical management, and results after extraperiorbital implantation of Silastic block, Br J Ophthalmol 74:545-550, 1990.
9. Smit TJ, Koornneef L, Mourits MP, Groet E, Otto AJ: Primary versus secondary intraorbital implants, Ophthalmic Plast Reconstr Surg 6:115-118, 1990.
10. Smith B, Bosniak SG, Lisman RD: An autogenous kinetic dermis-fat graft orbital implant: an updated technique, Ophthalmology 89:1067, 1982.
11. Smith B, Bosniak SG, Nesi F, Lisman RD: Dermis-fat orbital implantation: 118 cases, Ophthalmic Surg 14:941, 1983.

12. Soll DB: The anophthalmic socket, Ophthalmology 89:407, 1982.
13. Thompson N: Transplantation of dermis. In Converse JM, editor: Reconstructive Plastic Surgery, Philadelphia, 1977, WB Saunders.

CHAPTER 18

1. Andersen M, Vibe P, Nielson IM, Hall KV: Unilateral orbital floor fractures, Scand J Plast Reconstr Surg 19:193-196, 1985.
2. Becker FF: Surgery of the medial canthal region, Ann Plast Surg 7:259, 1981.
3. Callahan A, Callahan MA: Fixation of the medial canthal structures: evolution of the best method, Ann Plast Surg 11:242, 1983.
4. Converse JM, Smith B: Blowout fractures of the orbital floor, Trans Am Acad Ophthalmol Otolaryngol 64:676, 1960.
5. Dutton JJ: Management of blow-out fractures of the orbital floor, Surv Ophthalmol 35:279-280, 1991.
6. Goldberg RA, Lessner AM, Shorr N, Baylis HI: The transconjunctival approach to the orbital floor and orbital fat, Ophthalmic Plast Reconstr Surg 6:241-246, 1990.
7. Green RP, Peters DR, Shore JW, Fanton JW, Davis H: Force necessary to fracture the orbital floor, Ophthalmic Plast Reconstr Surg 6:211-217, 1990.
8. Heckler FR, Sonscharoen S, Sultani FA: Subciliary incision and skin-muscle eyelid flap for orbital fractures, Ann Plast Surg 10:309-313, 1983.
9. Manson PN, Iliff N: Management of blow-out fractures of the orbital floor. II. Early repair for selected injuries, Surv Ophthalmol 35:280-292, 1991.
10. McArdle CB, Amparo EG, Mirfakhraee M: Imaging of blow-out fractures, J Comput Assist Tomogr 10:116-119, 1986.
11. McCord CD, Moses JL: Exposure of the inferior orbit with fornix incision and lateral canthotomy, Ophthalmic Surg 10:53, 1979.
12. Nesi FA, Spoor TC, Ramocki JM: Management of blow-out fractures. In Spoor TC, Nesi FA, editors: Management of ocular, orbital, and adnexal trauma, New York, 1988, Raven Press, pp 321-335.
13. Nunery WB: Orbital floor fractures. In Levine MR, editor: Manual of oculoplastic surgery, New York, 1988, Churchill Livingstone, pp 201-208.
14. Patipa M, Slavin A: Axial dynamic compression plates in the management of complex orbital fractures via transconjunctival orbitot-

omy, Ophthalmic Plast Reconstr Surg 6:29-236, 1990.

15. Pfeiffer RL: Traumatic enophthalmos, Arch Ophthalmol 30:718, 1943.

16. Putterman AM: Management of blow-out fractures of the orbital floor. III. The conservative approach, Surv Ophthalmol 35:292-298, 1991.

17. Putterman AM, Smith BC, Lisman RD: Blowout fractures. In Smith BC, Della Rocca RC, Nesi FA, Lisman RD, editors: Ophthalmic Plastic and Reconstructive Surgery, St Louis, 1987, Mosby–Year Book, pp 473-490.

18. Raflo GT: Blow-in and blow-out fractures of the orbit: clinical correlations and proposed mechanisms, Ophthalmic Surg 15:114, 1984.

19. Smith BC, Beyer CK: Medial canthoplasty, Arch Ophthalmol 82:344, 1969.

20. Zide BM, Gelks GW: Surgical anatomy of the orbit, New York, 1985, Raven Press, pp 4-5.

CHAPTER 19

1. Bar S, Savid H: Lesion-oriented orbitotomy, Ann Ophthalmol 21:414-419, 1989.

2. Bergin DJ, Stewart WB: Lateral orbitotomy. In: Levine MR, editor: Manual of oculoplastic surgery, New York, 1988, Churchill Livingstone, pp 219-223.

3. Berke RN: A modified Kronlein operation, Trans Am Ophthalmol Soc 51:193, 1953.

4. Coulter VL, Holds JB, Anderson RL: Avoiding complications of orbital surgery: the orbital branches of the infraorbital artery, Ophthalmic Surg 21:141-143, 1990.

5. Jones BR: Surgical approaches to the orbit, Trans Ophthalmol Soc U K 90:269, 1970.

6. Kennerdell JS, Maroon JC: Microsurgical approach to intraorbital tumors: technique and instrumentation, Arch Ophthalmol 94:1333, 1976.

7. Krohel GB: Orbital surgery. In Smith BC, Della Rocca RC, Nesi FA, Lisman RD, editors: Ophthalmic plastic and reconstructive surgery, St Louis, 1987, Mosby–Year Book, pp 1084-1099.

8. Leone CR: Surgical approaches to the orbit, Ophthalmology 86:930, 1979.

9. Maroon JC, Kennerdell JS: Lateral microsurgical approach to intraorbital tumors, J Neurosurg 44:556, 1976.

10. Maroon JC, Kennerdell JS: Surgical approaches to the orbit: indications and techniques. J Neurosurg 60:1226, 1984.

11. McCord CD: A combined lateral and medial orbitotomy for exposure of the optic nerve and orbital apex, Ophthalmic Surg 9:58, 1978.

12. Smith B: The anterior surgical approach to orbital tumors, Trans Am Acad Ophthalmol Otolaryngol 70:607, 1966.

13. Smith JL: Anterolateral approach to the orbit, Trans Am Acad Ophthalmol Otolaryngol 75:1059, 1971.

14. Spoor TC: Anterior orbitotomy. In Levine MR, editor: Manual of oculoplastic surgery, New York, 1988, Churchill Livingstone, pp 209-217.

15. Wolfley DE: The lid crease approach to the superomedial orbit, Ophthalmol Surg 60:1226, 1985.

16. Wright JE: The role of surgery in the management of orbital tumors, Mod Probl Ophthalmol 14:553, 1975.

INDEX

Incisions(s)—cont'd
  full-thickness vertical, horizontal lid laxity
     corrected by, 138
  for gold weight implantation, 194
  for horizontal shortening of lower lid, 130
  horizontal tarsoconjunctival, sutures used for
     closure of, 138
  for injuries involving medial canthal tendon,
     50
  lateral canthal, closure of, 66
  for lateral canthal reconstruction, 92
  for lateral orbitotomy, 244
  for lazy-T correction, 134
  in lower-lid blepharoplasty, 146
  for medial canthal reconstruction, 96, 98
  for Mustardé technique, 82
  for naso-orbital fractures, 234
  parallel, for linear advancement flap, 18
  for preparation of conjunctival flap, following
     pterygium dissection, 210
  for revision of vertical shortening of lower lid,
     38
  for revision of vertical shortening of upper lid,
     36
  size of, in upper-lid blepharoplasty, 142
  for socket reconstruction, 214
  subciliary
    in reattachment of lower-lid retractors, 120
    reducing orbital blow-out fracture through,
      230
  subciliary blepharoplasty, 106
  used to locate superficial heads of pretarsal
     muscle, 50
  supratarsal crease, in external levator
     resection, 174
  for suspension of herniated lacrimal gland,
     152
  for temporal advancement flaps, 84
  for temporal transposition flaps, 86
  for transconjunctival graft from upper lid, 98
  for transverse blepharotomy and marginal
     rotation, 114–116
  for Z-plasty, 22
Integument; *see also* Skin
  anatomy of, 4
Intubation, canalicular, 48

K

Keratopathy, exposure, size of tarsorrhaphy
    determined by severity of, 192

L

Lacerations
  canalicular, repair of, 46–48
  lid margin, 44
  noncomplex, closure of, 16

Lacerations—cont'd
  transmarginal lid, lacrimal system ruptures
    and, 46
Lacrimal glands
  anatomy of, 151
  herniated, suspension of, 152–154
  palpebral portion of, excision of, 151
  surgery of, 151–154
Lacrimal system, 6
  dacryocystorhinostomy of, 157–164
  evaluation of, 1–2
  restoring integrity of, following transmarginal
    lacerations, 46–48
Lagophthalmos, 167
  Z-plasty for, 24
Lamellae, advanced, suturing, 202
Lateral canthal tendon plication, 28
Lazy-T correction, lower lid ectropion associated
    with frank punctal eversion repaired with,
    134–138
Levator aponeurosis, 6
  advancement of, in ptosis, 180–184
  resection of, in ptosis, 174–178
Levators, evaluation of function of, 167
Lid crease, re-formation of, in external levator
    advancement, 184
Lidocaine, in upper-lid blepharoplasty, 144
Lids; *see* Eyelids

M

Magnetic resonance imaging, preoperative, 2
Marcus Gunn phenomenon, ptosis and, 167
Maxilla, frontal process of, 8
Medial canthal tendon, 50
  repair of, 50
Motility, evaluation of, 1
Mucotome, Castroviejo, buccal mucous
    membrane graft obtained with, 112
Mucous membrane
  buccal, pedicle flaps lined with, 88
  pedicle flaps lined with, 88–90
Muscle
  preseptal, 6
  pretarsal, locating superficial heads of, 50
Mustardé technique, upper eyelid repair with, 82

O

Ointment, antibiotic, used on free skin graft, 36
Ophthalmic examination
  prior to blepharoplasty, 142
  preoperative, 1
    of ptosis patient, 167
Ophthalmoscopy, direct and indirect,
    preoperative, 1
Optic foramen, 8

Suture(s)—cont'd
  for base-down-triangle resection, 104
  buried, 14
  buried interrupted subcutaneous, 16
  chromic, 38, 122
    used to attach mucous membrane grafts to
      Gelfilm, 88
    used to close donor site, 36
    free skin graft secured by, 76
    skin incision closed with, 64, 68
  chromic catgut
    conjunctival flap attached with, 210
    used for entropion repair, 202
    used for full-thickness mucous membrane
      graft, 204
    for posterior flaps, 234
    used for split-thickness mucous membrane
      grafts, 200
  for cicatricial ectropion repair, 132
  used to close composite graft donor site, 68
  used to close donor site for dermis-fat graft,
    222
  used to close en bloc resection, 60
  used to close inferior-crus cantholysis, 66
  for closure of horizontal tarsoconjunctival
    incision, 138
  for closure of lid margin laceration, 44
  continuous locking, 16
  for correction of elevated brow, 30
  for correction of horizontal shortening of
    lower lid, 130
  for correction of lateral canthus elevation, 28
  for correction of lid laxity, 128
  for correction of lower lid and canthal
    malposition, 28
  for correction of lower lid laxity, 28
  Dexon, orbicularis transplantation using, 110
  double-armed, for transverse blepharotomy,
    116, 118
  double-armed Polybutester
    in external levator advancement, 182–184
    in external levator resection, 176–178
  double-armed prolene
    with OPS-5 needles, 128
    orbicularis transplantation using, 110
  double-armed Vicryl, for buccal mucous
    membrane graft, 112
  end-on vertical mattress, 14
  Ethilon, closure of severed canaliculus with,
    48
  following excision of cicatricial band, 24
  figure-of-eight, 14
  Frost, used in medial canthal reconstruction,
    100
  inaccurately placed, 12

Suture(s)—cont'd
  interrupted
    in bridge flaps, 78
    closure of incision over medial canthal
      tendon using, 50
    donor site closed with, 210
    following excision of facial and brow scars,
      26
    lid crease re-formed by, 184
    for linear advancement flap, 18
    in medial canthal reconstruction, 96, 100
    orbicularis transplantation incision closed
      using, 110
    skin closure with, 94
    for temporal transposition flaps, 86
    for temporal wound closure, 84
    for transverse blepharotomy, 118
    Z-plasty closure with, 22
  interrupted chromic, incision for sliding skin
    flap closed by, 76
  interrupted Vicryl
    free skin graft attached to tarsoconjunctival
      flap by, 76
    sliding skin flap attached to
      tarsoconjunctival flap by, 76
  for lateral orbitotomy, 250
  lid margin closed with, 64
  for marginal wound closure, in temporal
    advancement flaps, 84
  mattress, in lateral canthal reconstruction, 92,
    94
  Mesilene, bone flap replacement with, 250
  for mucosal flaps, 164
  for mucous membrane–lined pedicle flaps, 88,
    90
  in Mustardé technique
  near-far, far-near, 16
    combined with interrupted sutures, 72
    donor bed closed with, 86, 90
  nonlocking, 16
  Novofil, gold weight sewn to tarsus with, 194
  for repair of full-thickness lacerations of lid
    margin, 44
  for repair of naso-orbital fractures, 236
  for repair of orbital floor blow-out fracture,
    232
  for revision of vertical shortening of upper lid,
    36
  for semicircular temporal advancement flaps,
    72
  silk
    lid margin closed with, 44
    used to stabilize composite graft, 68
  for socket reconstruction with dermis-fat
    grafts, 218, 222, 224

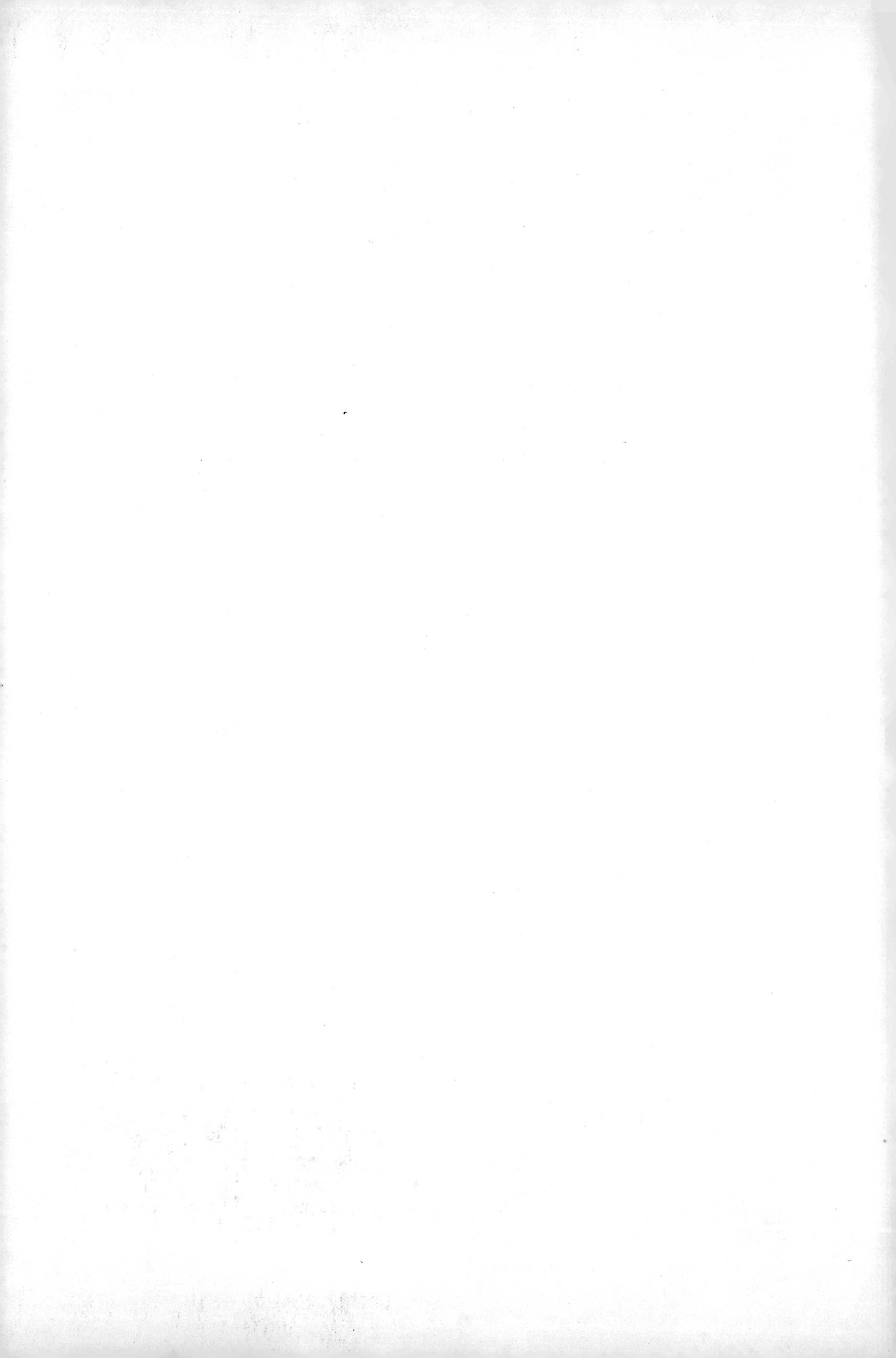